Mistletoe Therapy for Cancer

Mistletoe Therapy for Cancer

Dr Johannes Wilkens and Gert Böhm

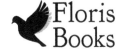

Floris
Books

An important statement

This book aims to contribute to a better understanding of mistletoe therapy and its potential for the treatment of cancerous diseases. The information it contains was carefully researched by the authors and is based in part on many years of clinical practice, and on the current state of scientific knowledge.

The applications and case studies described in the book are not intended for self-diagnosis and self-help, and cannot replace the advice and treatment of a medical specialist.

For a correct diagnosis and appropriate treatment in the case of health problems, or suspected or existing disease, you should always seek out a physician who understands the use of mistletoe therapy in individual cases.

Translated by Peter Clemm

First published in German under the title *Misteltherapie bei Krebs: Die sanfte Revolution* by Verlagsgruppe Random House GmbH in 2006
First published in English by Floris Books in 2010
Second printing 2018

© 2006 Kösel-Verlag, Verlagsgruppe Random House GmbH, Munich
This translation © Floris Books 2010

British Library CIP Data available
ISBN 978-086315-739-4
Printed by Lightning Source

Contents

Preface

New approaches in cancer therapy are not only desirable for patients but are urgently needed to reduce the costs of healthcare. Researchers and doctors throughout the world are feverishly working on new and better treatments; however, the hoped-for victory over cancer using only conventional medical methods looks unlikely — at least, there are currently no indications for such a success. Furthermore, the ageing population makes this problem increasingly urgent as the disease occurs predominantly after the age of sixty.

Many people do not take the danger of developing cancer seriously enough. But while its causes are still very much in the dark, most of the risk factors which favour the development of carcinoma have long been known: smoking brings about lung cancer; too much sun destroys the skin; an excess of alcohol leads to cancer of the liver; poor eating habits and unhealthy foods damage the stomach and intestinal tract; stress and a hectic lifestyle weaken the body's defences. Those with a hereditary disposition towards cancer are more at risk of the disease developing.

Most people know these dangers and they ignore them, yet much suffering could be avoided by conscious preventative measures against cancer. It gives one pause to see the many millions who nourish themselves with ready-made foods and French fries, flavour enhancers and additives, and to see cigarette smokers and the growing numbers of inactive, obese children. Too many people are not prepared to make preventative measures a part of their lives.

A sensible lifestyle is the most effective way to avoid cancer in the long-term; a second measure is through its early recognition.

Regular examinations have already saved the lives of millions of men and women, because malignant tumours were discovered at a very early stage. The chances of a cure are then high.

Besides prophylaxis and early discovery, there is currently great hope in a development that is still decisively rejected by many researchers and doctors: the bringing together of both old and new knowledge in the area of healing. It is perhaps from the combination of rich experiential knowledge with the great successes of modern medicine that the greatest advances in the fight against cancer will come. We shall see.

Indeed, mistletoe therapy, which has its roots in anthroposophy, is today a method which leads the way: in modern cancer therapy in Germany it is already used as a supplementary treatment in two out of three cases, and this combination of conventional medical know-how and anthroposophical insight works as a blessing for the patient. In our book we shall thoroughly examine the successes achieved by mistletoe therapy, right up to the thesis that this method is even suitable for prophylactic 'inoculation'* against cancer.

Sections in italics are direct quotes from and original citations of Dr Johannes Wilkens experiences.

---

* 'Inoculation' is not here meant in the usual sense, but refers to a special mixture of active ingredients that is injected into the patient at certain intervals. See also Chapter 7, Mistletoe Inoculation Against Cancer.

1. The Loss of Life Rhythm

Every epoch has its predominant illnesses. They result from the behaviour and attitudes of the people at that time — from nutrition and hygiene all the way to the inherent value systems and spirituality. In the current transition from the industrial age to the information society, the 'modern' man bears the stamp of materialistic thinking and actions to an excessive degree. The lack of love and warmth, and increasing egotism, bring about physical and mental illnesses that are typical of life becoming externalized. Cold or broken hearts can lead to heart attacks and other coronary ailments; stress, aggressiveness and the extreme tempo of life are ever more frequently transformed in the body into malignant tumours, in which the degenerate cells run rampant.

Our modern societies seem to be breeding grounds for these 'diseases of civilization,' which never before existed in such tremendous numbers. The occurrence of cancer in society is a reflection of the aggressions and incessant development of life. Many people seem to have lost their sense of moderation, their basic life rhythm is destroyed, they nourish themselves badly and live without a proper balance between sleeping and waking, between keeping still and moving, between tension and relaxation, and between work and rest. Many no longer take responsibility for their own lives but let themselves be steered almost entirely by their material wishes and cravings.

This one-sided attitude is dangerous because it forgets something of great importance: namely, that the organs in the human being, with their different functions, the combinations of cells and individual cells, are related to each other in impenetrable but wonderful ways. Body, soul and spirit are a complete work of art in life, in which everything is interlaced and woven together. Whether they are the tiniest body cells, feelings, or the fascinating mutual interaction of a universal order — everything is related to everything else; the entire human being is entwined in the great interconnections of creation. Therefore it is imprudent to treat cancer patients merely by focusing on their tumour, instead of expanding the view to include the whole human being.

At the beginning of the twentieth century, statistics on causes of death showed cancer to be in seventh place in Europe; today malignant tumours, together with heart and circulation illnesses, are at the top of the list. Due to increasing life-expectancy in the western world, and the prediction that people will nourish themselves even more unhealthily in the future, it is feared that the number of new cases will continue to rise drastically. Experts predict a likely increase of fifty per cent in these illnesses over the next twenty years.

In Germany around 400,000 people are diagnosed with cancer every year, predominantly with cancer of the intestinal tract, the chest, lungs and prostate. But however serious the diagnosis may be in individual cases, cancer is no longer a death sentence! Today almost half the patients can hope to be healed or to live for many years, thanks both to early recognition and because ever more men and women are prepared to undergo regular examinations. That is to be welcomed, but is still unsatisfactory, since most people expect more from our great science of medicine: 200,000 deaths every year from cancer in Germany alone are simply too many.

In view of the billions invested in research and the development of new therapies, the success of oncologists seems rather modest. With the help of surgery, radiation and increasingly controversial chemotherapies, modern medicine in many cases wins the battle against cancer; but there is no sign of a significant breakthrough, or an elimination of the disease. In addition these modern cancer therapies are almost always accompanied by serious side effects for the patient. With chemotherapy and radiation people often go through living hell: they lose their appetite and their hair, they suffer from vomiting, diarrhoea, constipation and depression. Their quality of life is reduced dramatically because their immune system has broken down.

But it's not just the physical suffering that torments the patient; cancer is more than 'just' a tumour. For most people with a carcinoma, their world suddenly falls to pieces. They descend into a black hole and can no longer escape from the terrifying thoughts: how far advanced is the cancer in me? Have metastases already been formed — in the lungs, in the head, in the intestines? Is there any chance of a cure? How long do I have to live?

In those first days following diagnosis, in which people are in a state of shock, they have to decide whether they agree with the method of treatment recommended by the doctor. What else can they do but accept the advice of the doctor? And with this begins a period of suffering, which is also accompanied by a kind of stigmatization of their life. People who during the chemotherapy or radiation treatment become emaciated and lose their hair often suffer more from this stigma than from the physical pain. Relationships with friends, acquaintances and fellow workers can change from one day to the next, because they don't know how to deal with the new situation. When they meet, should the topic of cancer be avoided, or is it better to speak openly about it? Should they speak about death, about pain with the afflicted person or should they steer the conversation towards more harmless topics?

So it's no wonder that old acquaintances and friends withdraw out of fear they might react in the wrong way. But for people with cancer this withdrawal leads to isolation, in which the now so urgently needed self-healing forces struggle to develop. A devilish dance begins, and in the continual mood swings between high and low patients can often lose their rightful hope for healing.

In the history of humankind, all former epidemics arose because bacteria and viruses entered the body from outside and destroyed it. With prophylactic inoculations the doctors could specifically target many viral infections and prevent the outbreak of fatal diseases. But with cancer the hostile instigator does not penetrate the body from outside, but arises within the human being and weakens the immune system. Poor diet, too little movement, stress at work and in one's private life evidently transform themselves in the human body in still unknown ways into a highly explosive mixture, which attacks the cells and leads to damage and degeneration.

A look at the history of medicine shows that the great pestilences of humanity —smallpox, the plague, leprosy, cholera, typhus, dysentery, tuberculosis, infantile paralysis, syphilis, etc. — could be controlled with hygienic measures and inoculation, and many of them have been entirely eliminated. And so at a time of highly developed medicine and technical equipment the question is: why is it not yet possible to overcome cancer by means of inoculation?

And so here we come to the topic of this book. It is in this respect that our experience and knowledge of the healing power of mistletoe can, above all else, open the door to a new kind of cancer treatment. This 'magic plant' probably provides the most hopeful direction for overcoming suffering from cancer. In conventional medical practice mistletoe preparations are being successfully used as a supplementary therapy against carcinoma. The currently available mistletoe inoculation, which is already applied to some extent, may soon, if used on a broader basis, be able to prevent the outbreak of a cancer epidemic.

Research laboratories have reported many times that an inoculation against cancer would soon be found. However, these hopes remain unfulfilled. That may be in part due to the fact that the substances used in inoculations can cause dangerous side effects; usually time-consuming research and clinical studies are necessary before inoculations can be carried out on human beings. With such a complex disease configuration as cancer, these preliminary procedures are particularly difficult. And so a preventative inoculation based on the principles of mistletoe therapy could become significant; the mistletoe preparations that have proved to be successful in the battle against cancer have already been proven to have no harmful side effects. People who are more at risk from developing cancer can now undertake short-term preventative mistletoe therapy, equivalent to a single inoculation, which can prevent the later outbreak of the disease.

In this book we aim to strengthen people's confidence in the healing power of mistletoe without giving exaggerated or false hopes to people who are suffering from cancer. The mistletoe therapy developed further by me has greatly helped the patients in our clinic, and has encouraged me to document this method inclusively in my inoculation thesis and to introduce it publicly. My professional medical reports and my lectures at medical congresses have produced a variety of reactions, ranging from enthusiastic approval to total and often malicious rejection, primarily from the ranks of conventional oncologists. But I am convinced that my 'optimized mistletoe therapy' and the inoculation thesis derived from it indicate new directions in the ongoing battle against cancer, and will hopefully soon find broad acceptance in medical practice — perhaps following the course of many new discoveries: first it is ridiculed, then it's despised, and finally put to use.

What can be done?

When someone is confronted with the diagnosis 'cancer' the question immediately arises: What can be done now? What course of treatment should I agree to take? In what do I have the most confidence?

The first and most important aim of conventional cancer treatment is the destruction of the tumour. For that there are the three 'classical' methods: steel (scalpel), beam (radiation) and chemo (chemotherapy); often they are also combined together, paired or applied sequentially. Further methods have recently been developed within conventional medicine that increase survival chances, above all with stem cell and hormone therapy. There are also hopeful beginnings based on the knowledge of immunology, above all a therapy with monoclonal antibodies which can inhibit the growth of the tumour.

As already mentioned, conventional medicine achieves its successes exclusively on the basis of ever improving methods of diagnosis and therapy, in laboratories and at the seat of the disease. But this detailed view of the tumour only reflects a restricted picture of the disease, because the occurrence of cancer involves the whole human being, not only the body. Therefore an expanded holistic treatment would substantially increase the chances of a cure. However, standard medicine is on a good path in its fight against cancer. But it could be even more successful if it did not limit its methods to just treating the patient's body, but also quite consciously included non-material aspects, in the sphere of the feelings and the spirit, in the recovery process.

Alternative and supplementary cancer therapies do this. From the age-old medical science of Tibet to anthroposophical medicine, all holistic systems of healing have one thing in common: they look upon disease as a disturbance that affects the soul and the spirit as well as the body. In view of this connection a fundamentally different understanding of the occurrence of cancer is required. The human being is a being in which bodily, emotional and spiritual states are knitted together in a complicated pattern of relationships. Although it's often difficult to trace the connections between these three levels, everything seems to be connected with everything else: the organs with thinking, feelings with cells, brain activity with heart attacks and breast cancer.

When an illness arises in a human being in one of the three levels, then that also has consequences in the other two. Therefore to heal means not only to treat the bodily ailments, but to work towards the recovery of the whole human being.

Throughout medical history the human being was always regarded as a unity; a separation between body, soul and spirit did not exist. Interestingly enough, at the present time ever more researchers, doctors and pharmacists of the scientific avant-garde are leaning towards this view, and the use of new methods in cancer treatment is going far beyond the one-dimensional approach of conventional medicine. The best-known methods in the holistic treatment of cancer are to be found in anthroposophical medicine (mistletoe therapy), in homeopathy, in traditional Chinese medicine (TCM), in physiotherapy, in hyperthermia therapy, in enzyme therapy and in the so-called self-regulation method. In the Appendix we have listed and briefly described the most commonly used cancer therapies.

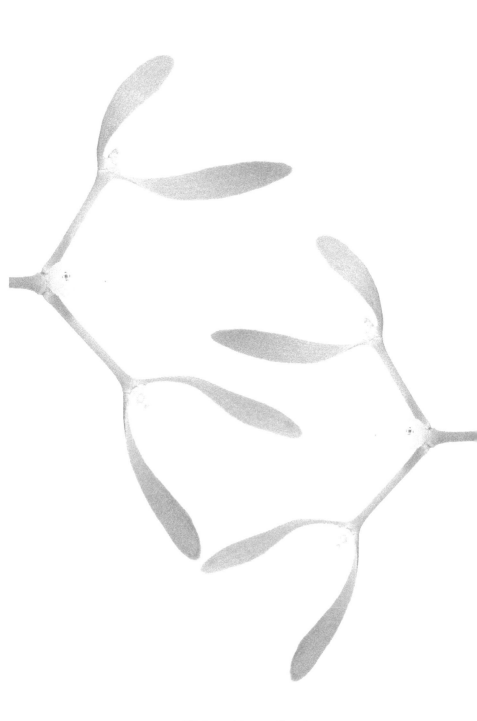

Mistletoe (viscum album)

2. The Key Role of Mistletoe

An introduction to mistletoe therapy

Together with conventional medical treatments, mistletoe therapy is probably the most significant method for overcoming cancer in the future.

Mistletoe therapy came out of anthroposophical medicine, which had its origin with the Austrian spiritual scientist Rudolf Steiner (1861–1925) and today has clinics and institutions throughout the world. Steiner's approach is very simple: based on classical, natural scientific medicine, it supplements its methods with spiritual scientific knowledge concerning the soul and the individual personality of the human being. According to the principles of anthroposophic medicine, both approaches belong together. Consequently it is not 'alternative medicine' but a complementary system of healing. Anthroposophical medicine uses everything provided by scientific research — medical techniques, laboratory tests, medications, operations and intensive medicine. But it goes a step further by taking into account the state of a person's soul — through speech, movements, emotional state, and in the most important life rhythms such as respiration, eating and digestion, sleeping and waking, tension and relaxation.

The anthroposophical physician lets himself be guided by scientific knowledge in his treatment of cancer patients, but in addition he also considers the psychological and emotional state of his patient — always with the aim of strengthening the patient's life forces. In this the patient is not merely the object of medical skill, but is a self-responsible partner of the doctor.

There is great variety in the therapeutic approach: it includes music, painting, conversational therapies, relaxation procedures, changes in diet and an ordering of one's way of life.

Of course the anthroposophical physician will also prescribe allopathic medications in cases of acute or life-threatening illnesses, just like his conventional medical colleague, but if that can be avoided he proceeds in a gentler way. In choosing anthroposophical remedies the attention is above all paid to stimulating the self-healing forces of the human being. This most often happens with natural, plant-derived, often homeopathic remedies, which act on the patient's soul condition as well as on the tumour.

The conventional physician selects medicines solely on the basis of scientific findings. The anthroposophical physician, on the other hand, tries to discover the 'relationship' between the sick person and the medication. The patient therefore must carry within his soul-spiritual condition a similar underlying pattern as the plant whose active ingredients are set against the sickness.

To carry out this type of an assessment, one can imagine how comprehensively trained and experienced an anthroposophical physician has to be: he must perceive, understand and judge the patient in his physical and psychological condition, and at the same time recognize the subtle connections between the character of the illness and the special active forces of a particular plant. The true connection between the physical and soul-spiritual forces of the human being with the corresponding properties of a particular plant cannot be discovered with logic alone, but also requires intuition on the part of the physician.

The active substances in mistletoe are perhaps the strongest medication we have against cancer; from them, in 1920, Rudolf Steiner developed mistletoe therapy, which has since established itself widely as a supplement to the conventional treatment of cancer. Today in Germany, six out of ten cancer patients receive mistletoe preparations in addition to the conventional treatments. Clinical studies have proven that mistletoe extracts distinctly raise the quality of life of patients, giving them increased appetite and work capacity, improved sleep and a greater resistance to infections. A reduction in tumour size and increased life-expectancy has also been observed.

An extract is produced from the mistletoe's branches, including twigs, leaves, blossoms and berries, which is usually injected under the skin of the abdomen. This preparation can in certain cases also be injected directly into the tumour or given by infusions. The commonly used under-the-skin injection can also be administered, as with diabetes, by the patient himself. Soon afterwards a reaction is visible around the point of injection: the skin reddens, sometimes itches, swells slightly and becomes warm — a sign that the mistletoe is beginning to work. It brings about a kind of fever and irritates the organism, which in turn stimulates the patient's self-healing forces and strengthens the immune system. Within the tumour itself, the active substances in the mistletoe restrain the rampant growth of cancer cells; they can often reduce the tumour and sometimes even make it disappear completely.

One of the main advantages of mistletoe therapy is how exceptionally well it can be tolerated. There are no harmful side effects, like those that accompany chemotherapy and radiation treatments. So far, following mistletoe therapy, there have been no reported cases of changes in the genetic make-up, malformations or the development of new cancerous tumours. Stringent testing in compliance with strict international standards has shown that mistletoe preparations can be used without hesitation.

What's so special about mistletoe?

As a supplement to conventional medicine, mistletoe perhaps offers, now and in the future, the greatest chance of healing for cancer patients. Why is that?

When you think about it, nothing about this ancient plant is normal! It's distinctly different from all other plants. The most striking phenomenon is that it doesn't grow on the earth, but on trees, and instead of roots it has a stake-like feeler with which it anchors itself in the wood of its host tree. Through this feeler the mistletoe nourishes itself directly from the tree. Like every other plant, it would be quite capable of providing for itself from the sun and its own leaves and stems; but it does not do so and nourishes itself preponderantly from the host tree it has tapped into. Mistletoe grows like an abscess in the crown of the tree, which, due to the parasite, gradually loses its strength and dies.

It's also noticeable that the mistletoe does not grow from below upwards; it overcomes gravity, being the only plant to spread its branches out in all directions and take on a spherical shape. The leaves of the mistletoe develop extremely slowly and only drop off after two to four years — green and hardly withered.

Mistletoe only grows from April until mid-June, then it pauses and rests until Christmas. Only when nature is in its winter sleep does it blossom and bear its fruit, the characteristic white berries. In the centre of each berry underneath the transparent skin is an embryo that is capable of germinating. But this seed cannot germinate by itself; it's 'locked up' in the berry and cannot leave the leathery fruit covering without outside help. In Central Europe the seeds are disseminated by birds, especially by the mistletoe thrush. The birds eat the berries, and their droppings, which contain the mistletoe seeds, are spread across the branches of trees. From there, sunlight awakens the mistletoe embryo, which can then drive its feeler into the wood. But strangely enough, not every seed thrives on every bark, but always needs an appropriate host tree: fir mistletoe embryos need fir trees, pine mistletoe embryos need pines, and the same principle apples to deciduous trees. Only the broom is different: the mistletoe seeds from coniferous as well as from deciduous trees grow on it. And in order to create even more confusion, apple tree mistletoe is widely disseminated: you find them on birches, poplars, elms and even oak trees, on which, as a rule, mistletoe very rarely attaches itself.

In the universal order of nature mistletoe has therefore created a totally upside-down world for itself. It's no wonder then that this mysterious plant has always fascinated humans and features so frequently in the world's myths and legends. The old Greek legend of Asclepius, the god of healing, tells us that illnesses were cured with mistletoe from oaks. In the heroic epic *Aeneid* by Virgil, the Roman poet, mistletoe opens the gate to the underworld and makes it possible for the dead to return from Hades. Thus mistletoe stands symbolically for the victory of life over death.

This symbolism of death and resurrection is found even more clearly in Norse mythology. Baldur, the god of light and beauty, is beloved of all the gods. None of the other gods is his equal in wisdom, purity and compassion, so they want to protect him from acts of violence. The goddess Frigga makes all creatures take an oath not to harm Baldur. When Loki, the crafty one, who hates Baldur, hears about it, he tears off a mistletoe branch, makes an arrow with it and gives it to Baldur's blind brother who, deceived by Loki, shoots the arrow that pierces Baldur's breast. For the Teutons his death was the greatest misfortune ever suffered by the gods and humanity: thus the mistletoe bore the blame for the greatest of all disasters. Perhaps, today, mistletoe can contribute to modern mythology once more as a powerful weapon in the battle against what is currently our greatest destroyer of life and health — cancer.

The Celts also believed that mistletoe possesses special powers. For them mistletoe berries were above all a symbol of fertility, an almighty divine seed, a symbol which, presumably because of the whitish and slimy consistency of its fruit substance, reminded them of sperm. The Celtic priests, the Druids, brewed a magic potion from oak mistletoe, which they cut at certain times with secret religious rites using a golden sickle. This drink confered fertility, strength and healing on those who took it. The Celt's belief in the magic of mistletoe is described in the *Asterix* comics, when the druid Getafix stirs up his magic potion in order to endow the Gallic people with supernatural powers.

In the Middle Ages many Christians believed that mistletoe had magical powers. They wore crosses and amulets of mistletoe wood or, while praying, they let mistletoe rosary beads pass through their fingers.

In Europe, especially in the Scandinavian and Anglo-Saxon countries, an old mistletoe custom has been preserved up until now: at Christmas time mistletoe branches are hung on the door to bring good fortune, health, strength and the rich blessings of childbirth during the coming year.

In the sphere of healing, the famous physician Paracelsus accepted the ancient recommendation to use mistletoe to treat epilepsy, for which it is still used. In the twelfth century the Christian mystic Hildegard von Bingen used mistletoe to treat sicknesses of the liver, and in 1543 the recommendation to treat abscesses with mistletoe is documented in book of herbal remedies. Other uses were for alleviating cramp, lowering blood pressure, and folklore advised pregnant women to carry mistletoe on their body in order to ease their confinement later on.

How does mistletoe therapy work?

Until Steiner's discovery at the beginning of the twentieth century, this mysterious plant was practically unknown in the field of cancer therapy. It had apparently escaped the critical observation of physicians, scientists and researchers.

The possible applications of *Viscum album* (Common or European mistletoe), first pointed out by Steiner in 1920, were confirmed in 1938 by the research of E. Koch, who carried out experiments with over one hundred plants with healing properties. At that time he was looking for active substances that were better suited for the treatment of local cancerous abscesses than the remedies then in use, such as arsenic, mercury and caustic lime. Treatment with these materials did indeed lead to the destruction of local tumours, but it was always accompanied by appreciable damage to the adjacent tissue. Furthermore the tumour decaying by necrosis has seldom had a lasting healing effect on the patient, but always caused great pain. So Koch wanted to find a substance that would remove the tumour without attacking the adjacent tissue or poisoning the whole organism. Koch's investigations in fact confirmed what Steiner had proclaimed: that mistletoe clearly had powerful anti-carcinogenic properties. But another half century would go by before the thesis of Steiner and Koch was taken seriously.

Today mistletoe therapy ranks almost as a 'classic' supplement to the conventional treatment of cancer, although it's still criticized by many physicians who cast doubt on the numerous scientific studies now available. This may, however, be due these physicians' dissenting relationships with anthroposophical medicine in general, from which mistletoe therapy comes.

Other scientists and physicians — in ever increasing numbers — accept mistletoe therapy because it has proven to be successful. In Germany, Austria and Switzerland more than half of cancer patients are already being treated with mistletoe preparations, and confidence in this gentle method is growing. In spite of all the successes, it must however be admitted that many of the details behind how mistletoe extracts work against cancer are still unknown.

So far we know that the mistletoe preparations affect tumours in two ways: they directly destroy tumour cells or restrict their growth, and at the same time they stimulate defensive cells in the immune system, allowing the body to tame the carcinoma with its own strength and restore order and normal development.

In an as yet inexplicable process, mistletoe substances induce apoptosis in the cancer cells, thereby promoting their genetically programmed self-destruction. Apoptosis is part of the regulatory principle of human life: in a healthy body millions and billions of cells are constantly being renewed and the destroyed cells are removed by a natural process. Without this exchange people could not survive for long. Thus our genes are wonderfully programmed: a cell dead due to apoptosis removes its remains by itself so that the surrounding tissue is not affected. The opposite condition is necrosis, namely the death of a cell due to serious damage from poisons, too high a temperature, etc. With necrosis the dead cells remain in the body, leading to violent inflammations.

Cancer arises when apoptosis is no longer functioning: when a degenerated sick cell has lost the capacity to undergo a natural death. When apoptotic regulation becomes derailed, the cells that would previously have been separated out remain in the body and continue to grow. With chemotherapy or radiation, one attempts to restore the apoptotic reaction, a difficult and usually painful process. Whereas this is where mistletoe preparations can achieve wonderful healing results, as we know from innumerable case studies.

Although the particular events that lead to apoptosis are largely unexplained, what precipitates the self-destruction of the tumour cells is still a great mystery. Despite the many investigations that have taken place, it is still not clear why results are so varied and what is really happening when the tumour cells self-destruct.

So how can mistletoe help people to overcome cancer?

There are well over one thousand different constituents combined in the mistletoe extract. These substances frequently work separately, but also in certain combinations. What exactly these combinations are is entirely unknown, but most likely, the astounding healing power of mistletoe is concealed within the complex interrelations of the individual components. Furthermore the active ingredients gathered together in the mistletoe appear to be more powerful in their totality than in the sum of their parts. Even though there is still much to research, the effectiveness of mistletoe against carcinoma has long been proven.

It is above all the lectins (sugar-binding proteins) of the mistletoe that help against cancer. In plants these lectins act as a protective inoculation against infections and cold damage, and something similar appears to occur in the human body. However the lectin content in mistletoe is only about one per cent, and this fluctuates depending on the host tree, on the time of year and on how cold the winter was in which the mistletoe berries were growing. Recently there have been attempts to put 'markers' on tumour cells and then to introduce the mistletoe lectin like a magic bullet. Those that hit the mark are supposed to promote the sick cell's self-destruction.

After being introduced into the human body the numerous and very complex effects of change produced by the over one thousand mistletoe substances are interwoven in the microcosmic convolutions of cells, tissue and organs within the body. These cascades of effects and convolutions make it impossible (given out current scientific capabilities) to make clear assertions about the curative action of mistletoe extracts; at best one can make conjectures about it.

Cancerous tissue is also extraordinarily heterogeneous: tumour cells distinguish themselves in their rate of growth, in their tendency to metastasize and in their reaction when subjected to chemotherapy, radiation, hyperthermia and so on.

This impenetrable interweaving of changeable relationships has so far made it impossible for an in-depth understanding or explanation of mistletoe therapy, let alone for proof using a scientific model. Meanwhile, however, extensive clinical investigations of mistletoe therapies are underway, but for the most part they do not meet the requirements of conventional medicine. The pragmatic approach is simply that it works. Everything is based on systemic assumptions which in practice lead to astounding results, but ultimately are unscientific.

Spontaneous remissions

The term 'spontaneous remission' is when a carcinoma shrinks or disappears entirely. Spontaneous remissions are very rare, but that could also be due to the fact that they are less commonly recorded.

Spontaneous remissions are of course what every cancer patient and physician dreams about. They can occur together with unconventional types of therapy, with feverish infections, with an allergy, with the influence of hormones, for example in a pregnancy or birth, or with psychological experiences and changes.

In the case of spontaneous remissions, the body somehow manages to self-regulate the orderly destruction of cells once more — triggered by an occurrence, as mentioned above. Mistletoe extracts are ascribed with the ability to bring about such occurrences.

Especially numerous and striking are the spontaneous remissions connected to feverish infections. Here there could be a connection with 'mistletoe fever,' which occurs as a desired reaction to mistletoe therapy (see also p. 136). In this age where we frequently use antibiotics, feverish sicknesses hardly ever occur, so in the future spontaneous remissions associated with fever will become even rarer.

With regard to this, the following is also of interest: research has determined that an especially large number of cancer cases have occurred in patients who seldom or never suffered from infectious diseases, whether as children or as adults. These people had hardly ever experienced fever or raised body temperature — a lack which later can have fatal consequences; through feverish infections the body's own powers of resistance are raised. This is above all true for feverish in childhood like mumps, measles and chickenpox, but also, for example, for women with pneumonia and influenza. However, conclusions from such immune processes may only be drawn with reservation.

3. The Anthroposophical Basis of Mistletoe Therapy

At the beginning of the last chapter we referred to the significant role Rudolf Steiner played in developing anthroposophy, and mistletoe therapy that arose from it. Let's look more closely now into this background and into what moved Steiner to research mistletoe and the human being.

Mistletoe therapy for cancer was born on April 2, 1920 when Rudolf Steiner gave a series of lectures for physicians and medical students following his own studies on mistletoe. In the thirteenth lecture he discussed cancer and a therapy involving mistletoe. Steiner's theories were based on his own anthroposophical model of the human being, which besides the body also includes the soul and spirit. Similar to the old Hippocratic teachings, he saw the human being consisting of four areas: that of the *physical body,* the fluid body (Steiner calls it the *etheric body*), the *soul,* and the *self* or '*I*'. Very few structures in the human being are physically hard, something of which even doctors are insufficiently aware. Almost all of the body's processes take place in a liquid state, a gaseous state (the transport of oxygen, for example) or in warmth (without a regulated temperature there is no human life).

In this the etheric body plays an important part: according to Steiner it contains all the forces which guide the growth of the body as well as the lawfulness of thinking. Steiner saw the disease of cancer as the logical result of an etheric body that has become too inactive. When certain processes in the body or the soul of the human being oppose the ordering principles of the etheric body then it becomes slack. That can then lead to the formation of tumours in certain parts of the body.

The symptoms of a disturbed etheric body usually appear many years before the outbreak of cancer — they are signals that draw attention to a life rhythm which is out of balance: poor, restless, frequently interrupted sleep that no longer provides body and soul with adequate strength; digestive disturbances such as diarrhoea, constipation and intolerances to certain foods. The soul can also be the harbinger of a tumour: lack of feeling and inner bitterness; an increasing inability to relate to oneself, to other people, to nature and to creation; unresolved problems and conflicts; unexpressed feelings or depressions.

A carcinoma therefore has a long prior history, and in the end it must be recognized as the body's revolt against those forces that subordinate themselves to the laws of the external world and destroy harmonious rhythm within the human being. The tumour then cuts itself off from the basic organization of the organs and cells, and with its virulent growth leads a reckless life of its own.

Steiner compares this with an image from nature: the mistletoe also cuts itself off from the normal course of the year, rebels against nature and against all the rational laws of growth. Hence the nature of the mistletoe is often characterized as 'insane.' According to Steiner's conception, the functional process of mistletoe development is like the way a carcinoma arises in the body.

In his legendary thirteenth lecture Steiner said the following words about this:

There is no doubt the potentized mistletoe is what we must now have in order to replace the surgeon's knife in dealing with tumour formations. It will then only be a matter of being able to work in the right way particularly with the mistletoe fruit, but also in connection with its other powers in order to make a remedy from it.

Steiner recognized that mistletoe has an inclination for an egotistic life of its own and opposes almost everything that the organizational forces in the human being want to achieve, including the formation of new cells. Mistletoe attacks the etheric as well as the physical body to such an extent that it can lead to an attack of cramps. With other patients mistletoe brings about feelings of dizziness or heightened sexuality.

A central and frequently cited sentence in Steiner's lecture is:

It is a matter then of correctly combining especially the glue-like substance of the mistletoe with a grinding agent, and of gradually producing a highly potentized version of this mistletoe-like substance.

Steiner also points out that mistletoe substances should not be given to the patient as a single active ingredient or as a mixture, but above all in the form of a potentized homeopathic dose.

In another part of the lecture Steiner specifies the effectiveness of mistletoe according to the host tree. He sees a close connection between a particular mistletoe and the organs of the human body. Moreover Steiner is convinced that the characteristics of the host tree must correspond to the person being treated in order for the mistletoe to develop its full potency. He also brings metallic substances into connection with certain forms of cancer, for example he recommends a combination of the apple tree mistletoe with silver salts as a healing substance for all forms of abdominal cancer.

The three key elements of his mistletoe therapy were summarized by Rudolf Steiner as follows:

1. Pharmacologically the potentizing of the mistletoe's individual parts (especially the fruit) is important.
2. There are connections between the host tree of the mistletoe and the individual organs in the human body, which are decisive for the correct choice of mistletoe preparations.
3. The healing power of mistletoe therapy is increased when it is combined with metal therapy.

From theory to practical application

In 1921, a year after Rudolf Steiner's lecture, Ita Wegman (1876–1943) showed the first results of therapy using mistletoe. While she could not report of cures in the sense of medical science, she had found in all the patients an improvement in their subjective state of health. Insomnia and fatigue had gradually decreased, and after the injection a euphoria was usually observed in the patients: they had recovered the will to live. With patients in the final stages of cancer, the mistletoe treatment led to an alleviation of pain, which meant that Dr Wegman hardly ever had to resort to morphine.

The pharmacist Willem F. Daems discovered what was presumably the first case history documented by Ita Wegman on the use of mistletoe therapy. It had begun three years before Steiner's lecture:

> 1914: Frau W. age 56. Radical surgery due to mammary carcinoma.
> Metastases in the supra- and infraclavicular glands (at the collar bone) and surgical removal of these with subsequent x-ray treatment. Then utterly miserable with complaints of constant weariness, total insomnia and inability to work.
> About two months after this second operation, beginning of viscum treatment and after about 28 injections, complete recovery from all disabilities.
> During the next six years the patient was completely capable of working. In 1923 she was again treated with viscum and lived to a great age.

First indications for an inoculation against cancer

Dr Wegman discovered something else from her treatments with mistletoe substances. She determined that:

Those patients who through heredity (carcinomas in the family) have a tendency to develop carcinomas and begin to be sickly, complain about fatigue and insomnia, have stomach aches and begin to have the appearance of being old — although neither a tumour in an organ nor changes in the mucous membranes can be confirmed — for this kind of patient mistletoe treatment has an extraordinarily good effect. Consequently one can here speak of a preventative therapy.

A comparison of Wegman's experience with what Rudolf Steiner told physicians in his thirteenth lecture seems to confirm that, above all, mistletoe has an activating effect which strengthens the etheric body. According to Wegman's observations at that time it was not yet possible to dispense with the surgeon's knife. Interestingly, however, she attributes the preventative action of mistletoe against cancer — a conclusion which, for the first time, provides an indication for prophylactic inoculation.

In Chapter 7 we deal in great detail with this thesis on the basis of actual experience; inoculation against cancer using mistletoe preparations is no longer a utopian idea, but from an anthroposophical point of view is already a hopeful and realistic course of action in the effort to defeat cancer.

4. Mistletoe Therapy Today

If one looks at the mistletoe products currently offered on the market and the requirements made by Rudolf Steiner, one is struck by the fact that what are offered are mainly not potentized medications; the connection between the host trees and the individual patient is hardly ever considered; even more rare are efforts to increase the effectiveness of the mistletoe with a metal supplement. However, for a differentiated mistletoe therapy to meet Rudolf Steiner's requirements, all three of these were specified.

Although Steiner's requirements are currently only partly fulfilled, mistletoe therapy has developed over decades to become a blessing for cancer patients, above all as a complementary therapy alongside surgery, radiation and chemotherapy. But apparently its real possibilities have yet to be fully realized. The successes so far allow us to anticipate the curative power that could be awakened when attention is paid to the mutual relationship between the host tree and the patient, as well as Steiner's other specifications. When mistletoe therapy is optimized in this way, perhaps the currently unimaginable will become possible — even leading to an inoculation against cancer.

Case studies

In order to show examples of the healing effects of mistletoe therapy for cancer, we have selected a few of the numerous documented case studies.

Bronchial carcinoma (lung cancer)

A well-regarded university clinic reported the remission of a non-small cell carcinoma. An inoperable bronchial carcinoma was discovered in the right lung of a 68-year-old patient. Following a period of very poor general state of health and coughing up of blood, treatment with a mistletoe preparation was begun. After two months there was a definite improvement: a remission of the tumour could be observed. With further treatment using the mistletoe preparation the condition remained stable for a year. Then, when the general condition deteriorated, the patient was again given an intravenous treatment with high doses of mistletoe infusions. Thereupon the general condition improved considerably and there was a definite remission of the tumour.

After nine months there was another deterioration, also in the area of the right lung. High dosage mistletoe infusions were again given and again the patient improved. He has now been in a good general state of health for three years.

Pancreatic cancer

A 65-year-old patient suffered from an inoperable carcinoma of the pancreas, which metastasized into the liver. The clinic had given this patient a life-expectancy of three months. She received mistletoe therapy and the initially very high tumour marker was reduced to normal levels. Other characteristics of the tumour marker were also reduced, which indicated a remission; that is to say, a stabilization of the carcinoma. The patient lived for another eighteen months and had a normal family life until three days before her death.

No pain therapy was necessary — that alone is unusual for a metastasizing carcinoma of the pancreas, which belongs to those tumours that most often require powerful painkillers.

Pancreatic head tumour

In 1983 a tumour in the head of the pancreas was found in a female patient born in 1923. It was the size of two fists and had metastasized enormously into the region of the left liver lobe with further metastasis in the right lobe. It was decided that neither chemotherapy nor radiation treatment was appropriate because no appreciable influence on the course of the illness could be expected. The patient then treated herself with mistletoe injections every two days with increasing, then decreasing doses. In addition she took other anthroposophical medications. Using ultrasound a slight remission was observed after four months in both the pancreas and the liver lobes. The patient felt well, and in the next two years her general condition and state of health remained stable. After two and a half years the woman discontinued the mistletoe injections; her general condition promptly worsened and ultrasound showed that the tumour was growing again. So the patient restarted the mistletoe treatment, and after two months she was well again and she experienced a healthy gain in weight.

Four years after the first diagnosis, there was no further growth in the tumour. She continued to feel well, which is noteworthy, considering her original condition.

Colon cancer

A 33-year-old female patient was operated on for colon cancer. But subsequently a new tumour infiltrated the uterus and the vagina, whereupon post-operative treatment was undertaken with chemotherapy and radiation. In a computer tomography (CT) scan a year later, metastases in the region of the pelvis and urethra were found; metastases had also invaded the liver.

After one year this patient also began mistletoe treatment. She received infusions of forty ampules of an apple-mistletoe preparation once a week. In addition she injected three ampules daily of a second apple mistletoe substance under her skin. Two years later another CT scan was again made, which revealed no further metastases of any kind. Also the metastases in the lesser pelvis and liver were no longer to be seen. The overall health of the patient was extraordinarily good: she had gained weight, her quality of life had definitely improved and twenty years later the original morbid appearance of the patient could now definitely be described as good.

Breast cancer

Carcinoma were found in both breasts of a 63-year-old woman, and they had already attacked the bones. Numerous metastases were found in all the dorsal vertebrae and in the pelvic and upper thigh bones. The patient suffered acute pain, her freedom of movement was very restricted and she could hardly walk. The physicians began with mistletoe infusions. After two months of treatment her condition had already improved and she could walk longer distances, and after three months the patient was entirely free of pain and could walk well. Under further examinations no metastases were diagnosed.

Breast cancer and lymph node metastases

A 56-year-old female patient had metastasizing carcinoma. Also in the left side of her neck were lymph node metastases, which had appeared after the first conventional therapy involving mastectomy, chemotherapy and radiation. She refused further chemotherapy because she was not prepared to go through the horror of it a second time. In the course of treatment with a mistletoe preparation, within a year the lymph node metastases went into complete remission and the tumour marker levels were halved. The patient has not since developed any further clinically radiologically determinable metastases.

Breast cancer and bone metastases

A 41-year-old female patient with a mammary carcinoma had to have a mastectomy three years ago. Under hormone therapy bone metastases appeared the following year. These were treated with chemotherapy and other hormones, but the further growth of the bone metastases could not be stopped.

Two years after the last diagnosis several metastases were found in the cervical and dorsal vertebrae, in the forward ribs, in both shoulder blades and in the right pelvic bone. The patient had acute pain with every movement and was tied to her wheelchair.

A mistletoe infusion therapy was begun, which led to a definite reduction in pain and a noticeable improvement in mobility. The patient could take up her professional activities again, take care of her family, ride her bicycle and carry heavy shopping bags. After four and a half months of mistletoe therapy a control examination revealed that the growth of metastases had been halted.

Prostate cancer

A 44-year-old patient suffered from a prostate carcinoma. There were already bone metastases, but the man refused to allow conventional treatment to be carried out. Severe pain attacks in the lumbar region of his spine were treated with medication by several orthopedists.

The doctors carried out mistletoe therapy, resulting in the original high levels of tumour marker being lowered by 25 per cent; in the following year they were reduced still further. At the same time the patient was clinically healthy and had no more pain. However he refused to have a scintigraph (an examination using radioactive substances), but one may presume that no further tumour growth took place.

Kidney cancer

The diagnosis of a 56-year-old woman showed kidney cancer. The carcinoma on the left kidney was operated on, followed by radiation treatment. However the woman's general state of health continued to be poor. A year later metastases appeared on the bones, namely in the right ribs and the neck of the femur.

A mistletoe infusion therapy followed, which led to an appreciable improvement in her general condition. Six months later a CT scan showed a complete remission of the bone metastases, and until today, that is two years later, no further bone metastases were found.

Malignant melanoma (skin cancer)

A malignant melanoma had caused brain metastases in a 59-year-old female patient, which were surgically removed. But a few months later further brain metastases had developed. This time radiation was used on the carcinomas, but despite the radiation they remained and continued to grow. Then after half a year lung metastases were found.

The doctors carried out mistletoe therapy, which at first had no effect on the tumour growth. About one month later they began to inject the mistletoe preparation directly into a melanoma metastasis that was growing under the skin of the right shoulder. It resulted in a strong inflammatory reaction and pain. At the same time all three brain metastases went into complete remission. The local mistletoe treatment was continued, but two years later two brain metastases and a further skin metastasis again developed. Again mistletoe was injected into the skin metastasis, and again the brain metastases went into remission. In the skin metastasis the mistletoe did not work — it had to be removed surgically.

Today, four years after the beginning of mistletoe therapy, the outcome remains unchanged.

Lymphoma (lymph node cancer)

This case concerns a 34-year-old female patient with non-Hodgkins lymphoma. Although the woman had gone through seven different chemotherapies in the last four years, they resulted in only a temporary remission of the lymphoma of three to four months. The patient was considered to be 'beyond therapy.' She was introduced to three different oncological institutes to find out whether any further chemotherapy treatment would make sense. All three clinics declined any further therapy as not providing any hope of success.

In order not to burden the patient any further in what remained of her life there followed only one more treatment with mistletoe therapy. The woman was greatly troubled by hot flushes, itching and disturbed sleep — her condition was rated on a medical scale with the lowest rating of six (very poor). The tumour mass was primarily found as lymph node metastases in the region of the left shoulder and in one tumour that went from the left chest wall through to the heart and had already advanced to the outer wall of the heart.

After one year of mistletoe therapy the CT scan showed an almost complete remission of the tumour; in particular the parts lying within the chest had retreated. Three years later the situation remains the same and the patient is almost free of complaints; painkillers are not needed. The disease has not progressed and no further metastases have been found.

Cancer of the bladder wall

This case concerns a 49-year-old female patient with a tumour that had almost completely penetrated the rear wall of the bladder. The back side of the bladder had already grown together with the pubic bone. Because of great discomfort, radiation therapy was discontinued. Then she experienced considerable pain in the lower abdomen and around the coccyx. The patient suffered from frequent lack of bladder control and was no longer able to work.

After mistletoe treatment was begun, the pain went away. Within four months the patient's weight increased by 7 kg (15 lb), and four weeks later she was able to work again. Over the next eleven and a half years mistletoe therapy resulted in a gradual remission of the tumours and in a substantial normalization of the bladder condition. The patient was able to continue work for the whole length of time.

5. Optimizing Mistletoe Therapy — Matching People with Trees

Despite the successes so far achieved by mistletoe therapy, the possibilities envisioned by Rudolf Steiner have not nearly been fully realized. Anthroposophical doctors estimate that at present only thirty to fifty per cent of the possible effectiveness is actually being attained, so tremendous potential still lies in the development of mistletoe treatment.

But the results so far are already impressive, as shown by the examples in the previous chapter. Mistletoe extracts demonstrably activate the cancer patient's immune system and can stop or at least reduce tumour growth. The patient's quality of life is improved and usually the mistletoe acts to extend the lifespan. Mistletoe therapy almost always enables the patient to become more capable, gain weight and increases appetite. They once again have a calmer and deeper sleep and are less liable to get infections. The case studies also show that mistletoe lightens the patient's mood and often helps to relieve pain.

Each mistletoe therapy is of course a very individual treatment. The substances used, the dose and the timing of the medications given cannot be reduced to a uniform pattern, but change from one case to another. Therefore the course of treatment, the medication or the dosage is sometimes changed, depending on how the patient reacts to the medication itself or to a particular active ingredient of the mistletoe. Thus the knowledge and experience of the doctor is of great significance.

However, according to Rudolf Steiner, in order to optimize the effectiveness of mistletoe treatments we must expand the method in two important aspects: before beginning therapy, a typological relationship between the host tree of the mistletoe and the patient must be clarified, something to which up to now insufficient attention has been paid. Additionally, metal substances should be mixed with the mistletoe's active ingredients that have been selected for the treatment. According to Steiner, this combination can markedly increase the curative possibilities with cancer.

Consideration of both these factors will by far surpass the level of effectiveness achieved so far, and hopes of healing this epidemic will grow. The vision of a mistletoe inoculation to prevent the outbreak of cancer may become a reality.

We will now explain these important, but rather complex aspects, and will refer to the improved and refined procedure as 'optimized' or 'typological' mistletoe therapy.

Optimized mistletoe therapy is no longer simply a thesis, but is already used in cancer treatments, for example in the Alexander von Humboldt Clinic in Bad Steben, Germany, as well as in other clinics and in the practices of anthroposophical physicians. So far hundreds of cancer patients — of whom many were considered to be beyond therapy — have been treated following this procedure, mostly with extraordinarily good results. Of course, as with all new methods, there have been disappointments, but on the whole the results so far have been very satisfactory.

Of course every form of cancer must first be treated with conventional medical methods. But clinical experience shows that life-expectancy can definitely be increased by combining conventional methods with optimized mistletoe therapy. The cases documented up to now are not sufficient to measure up to scientific standards, but they open the door to yet unknown ways. Whoever steps into new territory can seldom prove at the beginning that his method is right and will stand up to subsequent proof, and that is true in medicine. It is vital that optimized mistletoe therapy should be included in a broadly-based study extending over an appropriate length of time, so that the curative results can be evaluated over both the medium and long term.

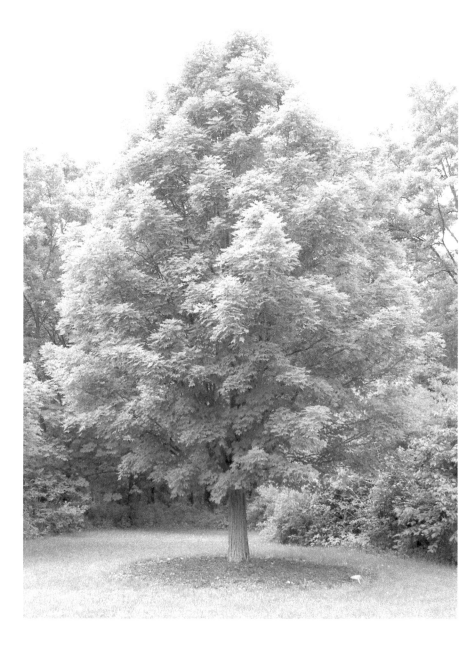

Field maple (Acer campestre)

When choosing the right mistletoe preparation, it is vital that the particular host tree matches the social type of the patient. This typological correspondence which, apart from my professional publications, is set forth for the first time in this book, follows from the analogy of tree and human being. For this purpose I have selected the thirteen trees whose mistletoe preparations are offered in potentized form by various producers today.

Each of these host trees has particular characteristics, which are described in botany, phytopharmacology, mythology and homeopathy, and which are also recognizable in certain human beings. Therefore I bring the attributes of the trees into a relationship with human types in the same way the physician Edward Bach (1886–1936) described them in his famous theory of the Bach flower remedies. He divided people into groups on the basis of their characteristics, without attaching any particular values to them, with all their strengths, weaknesses and individual problems. In order to make it more comprehensible I have outlined some of the character traits of trees and human beings more sharply, or consciously presented them in a simplified way.

The maple

The Latin family name of the maple is *Acer* which means 'pointed' or 'sharp:' this description refers to the pointed leaves. The fruits of the maple are often called 'nose-tweakers,' 'propellers,' 'helicopters'or 'little boomerangs,' because of the great love children have for them.

The sycamore (*Acer pseudoplatanus*) was also called the 'great milk tree' because its young branches contain a milk-like sap. In this sense one could regard the maple as the fig tree of Central Europe.

In Greek mythology the maple was looked upon as the tree of misfortune ruled by the demon of terror. In the *Iliad*, for example, the Trojan horse was constructed of maple wood.

In the Middle Ages, however, in contrast to antiquity, the maple was valued for its anti-demonic properties and used as protection against witches: pegs of maple wood were pounded into doors and thresholds to prevent witches from entering stables.

In 1424 in Trun on the upper Rhine, the Swiss Federation was founded under a mountain maple and renewed under oath every ten years.

To Canadians the sugar maple was so important that its leaf was chosen as a national symbol.

One could connect these last two thoughts with the fact that both the Swiss and the Canadians are renowned for being peace-loving and tend to be regarded as 'neutral,' making them less prominent in the history of the world. On the other hand, these two nations have the ability to effectively integrate different peoples and languages.

The maple is found in Europe, Asia, North Africa and America. It reaches a height of twenty to thirty metres, has a slim trunk and a thickly leafed crown which is usually egg-shaped.

Three types of maple grow in Europe: the sycamore, the Norway maple (*Acer platanoides*) and the field maple (*Acer campestre*). When its branches are injured the white milk-like sap oozes out; when badly injured, the trees can even 'bleed out.' The maple sheds the dead parts of its bark by itself. While the maple's blossoms are a favourite food for bees, it only blossoms after fifteen to twenty years. The long-stemmed leaf is typical, which, with its three, five or seven points, looks like an outstretched hand. The colourful splendour of autumn is caused in part by the gold-yellow leaves of the maple. The maple loves deep, limestone ground that is fresh and moist, but it has only a modest need for light. The leaves make good humus.

The maple is a favourite tree in city streets. But, surprisingly, relatively few people can recognize it from just seeing its silhouette but not its leaves — a sign of its insignificance, which is characteristic of the maple. The yellowish-white wood is elastic, pressure resistant and has fine fibres. It's used for making knife veneers, kitchen utensils, work tools and furniture, also for carving, and at one time for posts used in lake dwellings. It's a good wood for making musical instruments, for example violins, because it provides tone and resonance. For North Americans, above all the Algonquin Indians, the maple provided sugar, since the sap contains considerable amounts of sucrose.

Up to the present time, the maple has been valued in medicine, above all, as a wound dressing. It has a cooling effect, which reduces swellings, and serves as a remedy for persistent fevers. The maple's cooling properties reduce internal heat and distress, and rejuvenate tired, aching feet.

In traditional folk medicine the maple was also used for insect bites, swollen eyes and for liver ailments that led to digestive disturbances — quite in contrast to homeopathy, in which the maple plays no part.

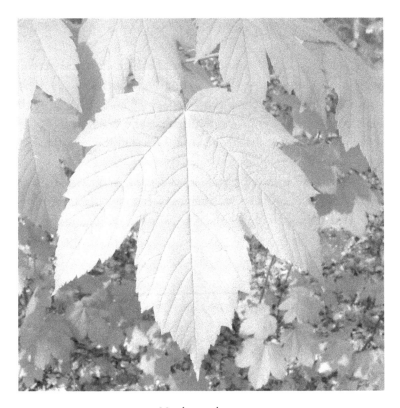

Maple-tree leaves

The maple person

The maple is the children's tree. It offers itself as a 'nurse' delivering sugar, as well as providing fun for children. Analogies to the human being are also demonstrated by its 'hands' and connection with music, since its wood is used to make musical instruments.

Maple people are modest, usually rather withdrawn, one can easily overlook them. They experience themselves as 'neutral:' neither blunt, nor sharp — therefore they go through the world without extreme, dangerous pendulum swings from joy to misery. Outwardly they appear altogether happy and give encouragement to others. They are often, themselves, good sounding boards for their own life situations: they can view many things through the eyes of childhood, and experience a newly won feeling of freedom and independence.

The maple gives self-confidence and helps restless and nervous people who tend to lose their inner balance in hectic everyday life; it helps them to become centred once again. It can restore the capacity for action in the 'modern man,' who tends to be guided through life by reasons in his head; it gives him the joy of making things with his own hands.

The special relationships between the maple and the human are relevant above all in pancreatic tumours, but also in cancer of the liver, carcinoma of the milk ducts in women and prostate cancer in men.

Pancreatic cancer

A 79-year-old diabetic female patient suffered from an advanced inoperable carcinoma at the head of the pancreas, therefore a combined treatment of radiation and chemotherapy was carried out. The very thin patient acted in a childish, naïve manner and was very trusting. She told of sharp pains in the upper abdomen after eating and had lost 10 kg (22 lb) in the last five months and suffered from the beginning of water accumulation in the abdomen.

The tumour located in the pancreas, the match between the maple and the patient's way of being — child-like, quiet, friendly and modest — as well as the pains straight after eating gave me direct indications for my decision to use maple-mistletoe, combined with a uranium-containing metal compound.

So in her very serious condition the woman received an optimized maple-mistletoe therapy; in addition she was given homeopathic medications and a platinum compound. While still in the clinic the patient's general condition was stabilized and strengthened so that she could be released. Her family doctor continued the optimized mistletoe therapy during the following months, with the result that although the tumour did not get smaller, the tumour markers were reduced to one tenth of their original value. In the subsequent months the size of the tumour remained unchanged and no metastases could be found.

A few weeks before her death the back pains returned strongly, for which only morphine plasters were of any help. But at the last examination shortly before her death, which took place one year after the beginning of the maple-mistletoe treatment, no metastases were to be found.

Cancer of the duodenum and the pancreas

A 45-year-old man had gone into a coma after a sudden lowering of his blood sugar. During the examination, tumours were found in the duodenum and the lower end of the pancreas. In the very difficult operation that followed, large parts of the tumour were removed.

Two years later the patient came to me. He was quiet and friendly, but very introverted. He spoke and complained very little. He mostly suffered from a painful pressure in the abdomen that occurred directly after a meal and spread out sideways. Every meal also caused him to have gas, his stomach felt spongy and his musculature was weak. Because of the location of the tumour and the matching symptoms with the maple, I decided on an optimized therapy with maple-mistletoe combined with a platinum metal compound.

After the first injection the stomach pains immediately lessened and after some time disappeared entirely. Meanwhile two years have elapsed since the start of the mistletoe therapy and the man's condition is stable. He is maintaining his weight and has neither pain nor other complications.

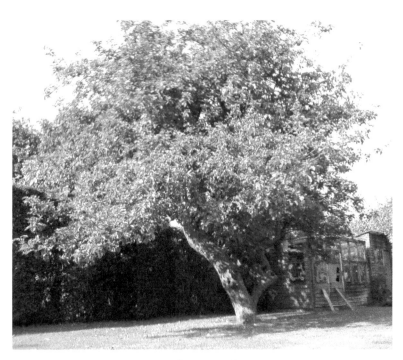

Apple tree (Malus)

The apple tree

The word 'apple' (Latin: *malum*, Greek: *melon*) comes from the Mediterranean and in the classical world described all exotic fruits that look like apples; small livestock, such as sheep and goats, were even called by these names. *Malum,* however, is not only the word for apple, but in the broadest sense it also stands for 'defect,' 'evil,' 'harm,' 'mischief' — in short, for what is evil (*malus* means 'evil' or 'bad'). Beauty and evil — the double meaning of the concept *malum* — gives the first indication of the ambivalence of the apple type.

The apple is one of the most common symbols in the world of mythology. From the very beginning there was a definite connection with the pair of opposites mentioned above: good and evil, harmony and conflict. In Judeo-Christian creation myth we encounter what is conjectured to be an apple tree. After Adam and Eve, despite divine prohibition, picked a fruit from the Tree of Knowledge, their access to the Tree of Life and thus to immortality was prevented. The bite of the apple got stuck in Adam's throat (Adam's apple). Eating of the forbidden fruit symbolizes on the one hand the temptation of evil, but at the same time it's a sign of newly won knowledge.

In Greek mythology the apple plays a significant and equally ambivalent role. It was a sign of love as well as — just as in the Bible story — an aspect of temptation. In the *Iliad*, the 'apple of discord' leads to the Trojan War. During a great wedding, Eris, the goddess of discord and sister of Ares, the god of war, angrily threw an apple with the inscription 'To the most beautiful' among the guests. Immediately a bitter quarrel arose among Hera, Athena and Aphrodite about to whom the apple should belong. The result was ten years of the Trojan War. Therefore the predominant symbolism, as in the Bible story, is of the fall into sin, into coveting and greed.

To the old Germanic ancestors the apple was an allegory of the mother's breast, of fruitfulness and nourishing love. In the late Middle Ages its meaning changed more in the direction of an allegory for original sin, but also as a symbol for might (as in the *globus cruciger*, the orb with a cross) and perfection. In the story of William Tell the apple is associated with the battle for freedom of the Swiss people, and in the tales of the Brothers Grimm both the apple tree and the apple play an outstanding role, appearing in twelve of the stories. In *Snow White* the apple shows its contrasting symbolism clearly with its white and red sides: one that preserves life and one that brings death. The story is also about beauty: 'Who is most beautiful in all the land?'

The apple tree is a member of the rose family, a plant family to which pears, quinces, peaches, apricots, rowan berries, wild plums, blackberries and strawberries also belong. They are all distinguished by their colours and smell, by thorns or prickles (for protection), by colouring or tanning properties, by essential oils, fruit acids, sugar and pectin, but also by poisonous substances from which, as from the almond, prussic acid (hydrogen cyanide) can be made.

Of the thirteen mistletoe trees described here, the apple is the only fruit tree. It appears small and compact and reaches a maximum height of ten metres (30 feet). Its outer form is distinguished by outspreading branches that project far to the side, and by a wide, densely-leafed crown. Both crown and fruit are round. On ground rich in limestone and fresh nutritious soil and in a sunny region, apple trees bear ample fruit. But areas with late frosts are less suitable for their cultivation.

The apple tree's wood is hard, dense and difficult to split. There is often a tendency towards twisted growth and it rots rapidly when exposed to dampness. But since it can easily be worked by turning, planing and carving, and can be easily polished and stained, people have always liked to use the wood for making toys, weaving shuttles, wooden screws, and as a veneer in furniture making.

The apple is one of the most beloved trees in Europe — no wonder, then, that it has a firm place in folk medicine and in nutrition (an apple a day keeps the doctor away). It aids digestion, but can also be constipating and promote urination. The fruit contains vitamin C, calcium, iron and pectin. Pectin can hold one hundred times its own weight in water and is used for making jam. A grated apple is an effective treatment against diarrhoea. In cases of bladder and kidney stones, a diet of apples helps to get rid of the deposited matter. It is said that tea made from apple peel calms the nerves and helps prevent a craving for fats. The bark of the root is supposed to be a remedy for diabetes.

The use of apple substances is not known in homeopathy.

In Bach flower remedies essence from the blossom of the crab apple, or wild apple, is used as a cleansing medication to help people who feel that something within themselves or in their environment needs to be cleansed.

The apple-tree person

Rounded, 'pomaceous' patients who feel unattractive because of their small stature are likely to have a relationship with apple-tree mistletoe. Often their skin is wrinkled, like the bark of the apple tree. These people are often very phlegmatic; their lethargy frequently affects their food assimilation so that they suffer from acute indigestion. They also have a tendency towards anaemia.

Apple-tree people are often critical of their appearance or of their personality, and are compulsively clean, feeling the need to constantly wash their hands or take a shower. They demand total perfection of themselves and their surroundings, and when these exaggerated requirements cannot be fulfilled they react with great confusion. At first this almost compulsive attitude takes the form of fussiness. Also 'oral fixations' (constant fear that there is not enough to eat) occur frequently.

In apple-tree people, carcinomas tend to develop in the lower digestive tract. Apple-tree mistletoes work particularly against cancers of the colon and liver, as well as in apple-tree women suffering from breast cancer, ovarian cancer and cancer of the uterus. For them, carcinoma of the bones as well as of the blood and lymphatic system are also typical.

Prostate cancer

A carcinoma of the prostate was found in a forty-year-old patient. He refused an operation and decided on chemotherapy, which did not result in any observable remission of the tumour. The diagnosis, which had been made eighteen months before, had completely thrown him off balance inwardly; he lived in perpetual fear that the carcinoma could spread to his intestines.

In a psychotherapy session many things that had been greatly burdening him came to light. For example, he came into the world with the umbilical cord round his neck. His mother had not wanted him, so in childhood the boy was often beaten by his parents. His mother also punished him by withholding her love, and always made it clear that she had no time for him.

At the age of 36, his whole body suddenly turned yellow, and he underwent a three-hour operation for a perforated gall bladder. Although he was completely anaesthetized, he was conscious of the whole operation and could later describe it in every detail. After the operation he also stopped breathing and had to be resuscitated (second birth).

He had an unhappy first marriage that ended in divorce. He appears to be content with his current partner. He's glad to be alive and can thoroughly enjoy himself, yet he tends to be dissatisfied. He is plagued by many feelings of guilt, due to his own imperfections as well as from being deprived of his mother's love and that of his first wife. He goes into a panic at the mere mention of love deprivation.

Because of his many feelings of guilt and shame, his thirst for pleasure and his rather stout build and pot belly, I prescribed an apple-mistletoe preparation for the patient. But because there are also choleric and powerful aspects of his being (twice surviving dangerous situations, his firm voice and his great professional ability) I also added an oak-mistletoe substance as well as silver and iron compounds.

After six months, the CT images showed no metastases, the enlarged lymph nodes had disappeared, the prostate had returned to its normal size. The patient radiated satisfaction and could now come to terms with his family history, living through a third birth.

The birch

The word 'birch' comes from the Indo-Germanic 'bak' or 'berk' (light, white). Because of the thin, drooping branches the white birch is also known as 'hair birch.'

The birch is connected like no other tree with northern Europe and Siberia. The white birch symbolizes the world tree for the Siberian Tartars, as the ash does for the Germans. For the Shamans it was the tree of life, which opens the gate to heaven.

Originally the birch represented the divine rebirth of the light. Since the fifth century the birch has had a special relationship to St Bridget of Ireland, who was seen as the Virgin beneath the trees. Purity and beauty are wonderfully combined in this unusual tree. The feast of St Bridget on February 1, the eve of Candlemas, symbolizes the inner and outer purification of the human being (linked to the Latin word *februare,* meaning to cleanse, to atone). The Christian festival of the Candlemas of the Purification of the Virgin has existed since the fifth or sixth century.

The birch has a slender, pliant trunk. While it lives to around eighty years old, its growth in height slows down perceptibly after twenty years. Birches, along with poplars, belong to those pioneer plants that brought nature back again after the ice age — no other leaf tree is so resistant to winter. The birch needs plenty of water, and as was previously mentioned, it needs light: it thrives poorly in forests. It has a flat root system and absorbs much nutritive material from the ground surface, leaving little for other plants.

Birch is hardly ever used for building. Its wood was and is still valued for the production of poles, clogs, barrel hoops, ladders,

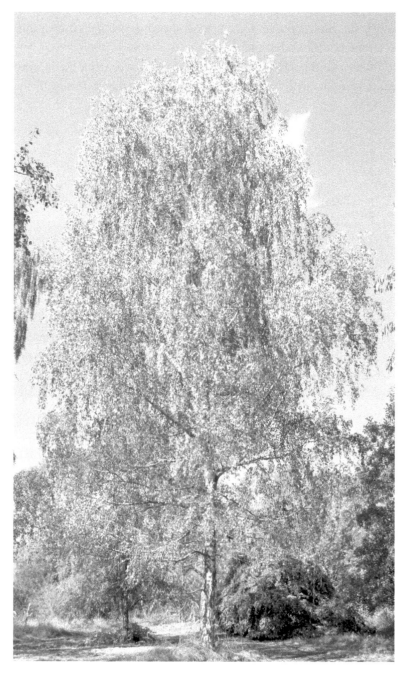

Silver birch (Betula pendula)

tables, chairs and clothes pins. The pitch which prevents wagon wheels from squeaking was also obtained from birch wood.

Brooms and switches were made from its branches, with which people whipped their bodies in Scandinavian saunas — as part of their inner cleansing routine.

People like to collect birch sap from older trees, and it's very popular as firewood because of the high content of essential oils and resins. The bark, which is used as an underlay for steep roofs and beams, also contains an important constituent — tannin — which was formerly used for tanning animal hides. In those days the bark was also used as a paper substitute.

In medicine, birch sap was formerly used to prevent the formation of kidney stones and jaundice. It was considered an effective remedy for oedema (dropsy) as well as gout, scurvy, depression, cancer and skin problems. Birch foliage was a proven remedy for rheumatism, gout and painful swollen joints.

The excellent effect of the birch for regulating water retention and for the treatment of people suffering from depression has always been highly valued in traditional folk medicine. According to arboreal medical practice, the birch brings light and joy into the soul and returns movement to a life marked by lethargy and rigidity. It can light up the soul after many bitter disappointments and bring back new courage and cheerfulness.

In homeopathy birch charcoal is used above all else, especially for older patients suffering from chronic ailments of the respiratory tract. However, when a person's life forces are dwindling, the active substances in the birch (*carbo vegetabilis*) also help to ease the dying process.

The birch person

The birch type, like the bark itself, is marked by the polarity of black and white, as well as by the strong relationship to light, which symbolizes purification. They are human beings who can deal with life and with death. Mostly they appear to us as light, bright people of slight bone structure, as lively, cheerful people with a sanguine temperament. They can quickly become enthusiastic about tasks and other people, but after the initial burst of flame they often lack the physical strength to bring ideas to realization. Work comes easily to birch people and because of their good communication skills they bring joy and light into the dullest of company.

Skin cancer has often been found in the light-skinned birch type. In women, carcinoma of the ovaries predominates, and there is a notable tendency for allergies. Birch medications are especially appropriate for patients who have lost their youthful buoyancy and feeling for charm and beauty in their life. When people can no longer feel happy and relaxed in a child-like way, are frozen within themselves and their life energy no longer flows, the doctor must consider birch mistletoe, usually combined with a copper compound. Birch is also the chief remedy for bladder or kidney carcinoma in women.

Breast cancer

A 43-year-old woman had a carcinoma surgically removed from her left breast. The operation went without any complications, and no metastases were found. This was followed up with chemotherapy. The patient came to our clinic for a further treatment with mistletoe therapy.

She was a thin, red-haired woman with a fine bone structure. She had a considerable amount of whitish, but also brownish-black pigmentation on her skin. The patient, who was a carer, told of feelings of utter powerlessness. Before the operation her libido had declined considerably. During this time she had felt exhausted, especially from the many night shifts. In springtime she always suffered from hayfever, especially from birch pollen. On the whole, the patient made an alert, almost cheerful impression. She was very much alive intellectually, and actively worked in the church community.

The woman's slight build, the white and dark spots on her skin, her allergic reaction to birch pollen, as well as her inclination towards social and intellectual activity were indications to me of an inner relationship to the quality of the birch. Therefore I prescribed a birch-mistletoe therapy for the patient, supplemented by a homeopathic treatment with phosphorus.

After the second injection she felt a definite increase in libido and generally felt stronger.

The third injection produced a violent fever of 40°C (104°F). At an examination a year later, the woman was feeling well generally and her hayfever had also gone. No further carcinoma was found and there were no problems with her vitality.

Skin cancer and metastases in the lung and brain

The relationship of the birch mistletoe to allergies is also shown in a very instructive case from the German oncologist Dr Broder von Laue. He treated a 56-year-old patient with a malignant melanoma (skin cancer). The melanoma had appeared in the neck, but disappeared again in a spontaneous remission. Three years later metastases were found in the lung and the brain and surgically removed. It turned out then that melanoma cells were involved.

As new brain metastases then developed, the ongoing radiation therapy was discontinued and a birch mistletoe therapy was begun. With this treatment slight symptoms of nettle rash and itching appeared shortly after the injection. At the same time the metastases in the brain and lung became smaller. In the ongoing course of intensive mistletoe therapy there was a total remission of the brain metastases and the lung metastases became smaller.

Unfortunately, in spite of the mistletoe therapy, a new brain metastasis appeared. This time a therapy with pine mistletoe was used, later also with oak mistletoe, and again there was a complete remission of the metastases.

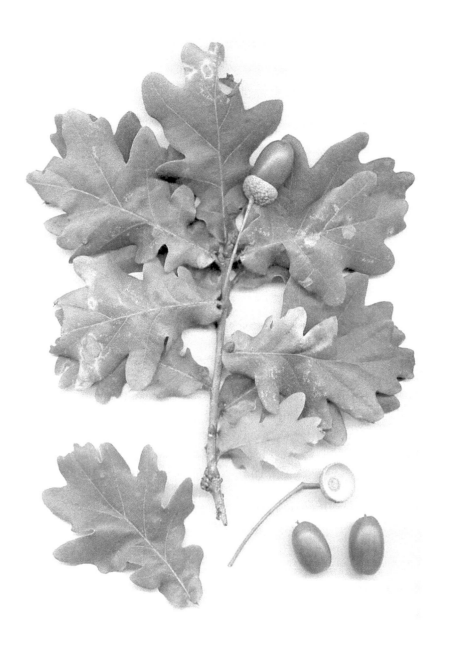

Oak-tree leaves and acorns (Quercus robur)

Later on a node started to grow in the right side of the neck. During the attempt to remove this metastasis surgically the patient died — six years after the first mistletoe treatment was begun.

The oak

In Latin the English oak has the name *Quercus robur* (*Quercus* means oak, *robur* means robust or strong). In Bavaria it is also called *Knobber-Oachen* because the oak brings forth so-called 'knobbers,' which are gall formations in the calix made by gall wasps. Even before the famous oracle at Delphi, there was a sacred oak at Dodena in Greece. The priestesses of this cult prophesied from the movements of the leaves. Greek mythology also tells us that divine connections were made between the oak and the mistletoe in this most ancient of Greek rituals.

The hills of Rome were originally covered with oaks dedicated to the god Jupiter. On Capitol Hill the first temple to Jupiter was built by Romulus near an oak that had long been an object of worship. On the branches of this oak Romulus hung the trophies he had taken from the enemy. After him, this was also done by the heroes of Rome, the *Imperators*, who climbed up Capitol Hill wearing heavy crowns of oak leaves. Rome was therefore always a place of worship of the oak.

The world of the Norse sagas is also unimaginable without the oak, in which it was the most revered of trees. The Celts as well as the Germanic peoples worshipped their gods not only in sacred groves and springs, but also in trees. Most well known is the Donar oak of St Boniface in Geismar (near Fritzlar, Germany). Donar was the lord of lightning. Later, during the course of Christianization, many oaks were cut down in order to demonstrate the powerlessness of the native gods. Nevertheless the cult of the oak was preserved in Germany. For the Celts, the oak was the most sacred tree, and the mistletoe which grew on it (oak mistletoe was and still is found very rarely) was revered in a special way. The relationship of the Celts to the oak is known popularly today through the tales of Asterix and Obelix.

Moreover, the oak was generally regarded as the tree of life; the tree which brings rain and regulates the circulation of water. The oak was not only seen to be nourishing, but also as promoting fertility. Throughout mythology the oak has been looked upon as the tree of fertility, of plenty and of social contact. The oak even became known as the thing tree, under which the thing — the assembly of free people — used to be held, and here a relationship to the lime tree becomes apparent. However, the lime and the oak differ in the impression they make and in their symbolic significance. Whereas the lime, with its heart-shaped leaves and sweet aroma, expresses the feminine, motherly principle, the strong austere oak stands for the masculine principle, for fatherly strength and severity. In this connection one may recall the pair of lovers of ancient mythology, Philemon and Baucis, who were changed into a lime and an oak tree.

The oak is not only the mightiest, but also the best-known tree in Europe. Oaks grow in slow steady fashion, some of them to an immense size. It forms gnarled, widely spread and often horizontally extending branches. It has a mighty crown with strong branches. Oaks grow to about 30–35 metres (100–120 feet) high, even sixty metres in exceptional cases. This imposing tree has a strong, deeply-extending tap root that holds it fast even in the most powerful storm. In its first one to two hundred years the oak gains rapidly in height; the following years are devoted to increasing its girth. Folk wisdom distinguishes between five hundred years of ascent and five hundred years of decline: in its youth, the tree has a smooth shining bark, brownish to light grey in colour, which later turns into a dark brown rind, full of rents and with a high tannin content.

Wild bees often live in the hollow spaces of the oak. It also provides a habitat for the woodpecker, for numerous beetles, other birds and up to a thousand kinds of insects; so in nature the 'social,' protective capacity of this tree reveals itself.

The benefits of the oak have been praised in many cultures, even the soft woolly balls made by gall wasps, which were used as fuel in lamps. They were also used in ancient times as a dye, for making ink and tanning leather.

Of all trees, the oak has the strongest wood. Historically warships were built out of four thousand oaks. However, oak wood cannot stand iron, which causes ugly stains on its surface. It has always been the most important wood for construction, both above and below ground, having been used for making barrels, railroad ties and inlaid floors, building canal locks, ship frames, floors, window sills and water wheels. Cork is made from the cork oak (*Quercus suber*).

The oak's acorns have always been used to feed pigs, but they were also used as a substitute for coffee beans.

In traditional European medicine the oak was used for infections of the alimentary canal and the bladder, as well as for catarrh of the mucous membranes and excessive menstrual bleeding. Oak substances served to strengthen the lower pelvic muscles and were used to ease varicose veins and haemorrhoids. According to other reports, oak also neutralizes the craving for alcohol. Baths with oak bark heal skin abscesses and, according to Sebastian Kneipp, the proponent of hydrotherapy, one should use oak preparations for goiters and swollen lymph glands. In folk medicine, the oak is used above all externally to treat eczema.

The oak has a relationship with the spleen and works as an astringent and drying agent. In the lumber industry it has been found that dust from oak wood can lead to tumours in the nasal passages. On the other hand, oak bark is found to provide a good remedy for catarrh and blocked nasal passages. It is recommended as a mouthwash for inflamed gums and mouth ulcers as well as a gargle for sore throats, tonsillitis and laryngitis.

In homeopathy oak is used as a medication for alcoholism; it strengthens a diseased liver. Liver problems, dropsy, gout and an enlarged spleen are the principal diseases that can be treated with oak substances. The curative relationship of the oak to the liver, as well as to rough, dry skin, has recently been confirmed by medical research.

The oak person

Oak mistletoe is useful for old, exhausted battlers, above all for patients who have had to work hard all their lives. They are the prime example of what society considers to be the attribute of 'manliness.' Oak people never permit themselves any weaknesses. Rather they are people who have always — also in a figurative sense — taken good care of their house and home, although their dwellings usually display a certain emptiness. While patients have good outward creative ability, there are often deficits in relation to themselves, above all in their own inner life of feeling, as well as a lack of consciousness for relaxation and fun. The oak analogy is often valid for farmers or people who have seldom left their little plot and only unwillingly go on vacation.

The being of the oak is above all found in patients in whom strength, persistence and a strong will is accompanied by high ideals. However, they tend to lead a rather rigid life and they put enormous pressure on themselves and on others to achieve and succeed. In a positive sense, one can describe these people as reliable, assiduous and faithful to their duty. Oak patients, however, never want to show that they are weak or no longer able to help others.

Oak people frequently believe that they are being somehow hard done by. They typically feel as if they are having to fight against untruths and are being dealt with unfairly, even to the point of believing that others will only be successful if they interfere. They give the impression that they are busy all the time, they become annoyed quickly and often, and complain a lot of being tired in the morning. Their inner world, the condition of their soul, is altogether reminiscent of the Old Testament. Their concept of morality is often strikingly black and white. They possess strength and reliability to the point of stubbornness.

The build of an oak patient gives the impression of being compact or athletic and they have firm, strong skin. They believe they will only receive acknowledgment in society if they achieve something special; that's why oak people count as good and effective workers. Therefore it's not surprising that it's primarily men who become sick with oak symptoms, and often in those organs which stand for manliness — above all in the prostate, liver and gall bladder. Otherwise bone tumours, leukaemia and cancer of the lymph glands are also typical of oak people.

Prostate cancer and tumour in the large intestine

A carcinoma was found in the prostate of a seventy-year-old man as well as a tumour in his large intestine. The patient had a strong, athletic stature, was mobile and dynamic and had clear ideas about his life plans. The carcinoma in the prostate was surgically removed. But after that he suffered constantly from back pains, although there was no bone metastasis. However, he did suffer from high blood pressure.

Because of the patient's overall agile condition, the fact that he was an athletic type and based on his very positive attitude to life, it was the oak which immediately occurred to me.

Therefore treatment with oak mistletoe was begun, and in addition he had to drink wild-rose tea containing iron. This treatment raised his body temperature to 39°C (102°F). The regular back pains that had persisted until then disappeared completely and the man could go walking again without any trouble. His previous continual need to urinate diminished and his weakened sexual drive rose again. Also the development of the re-grown prostate carcinoma was negative: when it was checked, no more cancer cells were found in a probe of the tissue, and what's more, a protective shell of inflammation had enveloped the tumour, which was no longer malignant.

Prostate cancer

One patient had radical surgery to remove a prostate carcinoma and the testicles. He had a vigorous personality, came from a family of farmers and had grown up on the land. He had had to overcome many blows of fate during his life: his wife had left him overnight and then demanded a lot of money from him; his son had been severely scarred by burns, and his granddaughter had been born blind.

The patient always felt too warm at night; he apparently generated too much heat. When he lay down in bed many severe cramps started in his legs, in which there were clear signs of varicose veins. Following the operation the man felt relatively stable and well, but after eight years the tumour marker again indicated a cancerous condition, and lymph node metastases were found in the entire abdomen. Following immediate chemotherapy a blockage developed in the intestines and in the connection to the gall bladder. Chemotherapy was discontinued and the patient received radiation treatment.

In this situation the man came to me. Based on the patient's biography and the many blows of fate that he had always faced with courage, I saw an analogy to the character of the oak.

Therefore the man was given an oak-mistletoe preparation, injected under the skin twice a week, in addition to which he was given a copper compound. Just a month later he felt — to use his own words — 'released.' He no longer felt so hot at night, the varicose veins in his legs had almost completely disappeared, and the leg cramps no longer occurred. The patient is once again happy and well. How long this will last is, of course, uncertain.

The ash

The name 'ash' is derived from the Indo-Germanic root 'os,' which expresses a close relationship to spring water; it is also part of the names of cities, such as Oslo or Osnabrück and emphasizes the ash trees appearance in the vicinity of springs.

Some of the folk names for the ash are also interesting from an etymological perspective. In parts of Germany ash trees are called 'bird tongues' because of the tongue-shaped fruit, or 'bow tree' and 'spindle tree' after the wood's common uses. Another name is 'wound wood' because ash supposedly has a healing effect when rubbed on wounds, and the name 'goat tree' came about because the leaves are used for goat feed. In Tyrol it is called 'tension wood' because it was used against loss of muscle tension.

The European or common ash's Latin species name of *excelsior* takes into account the shape of the tree: tall and majestic. It's a reference to the strong, deeply-rooted character of the ash, which grows up high and in the sunlight produces a magical display with its tender leaves. In the ash the desire to be great becomes visible, branches and leaves losing themselves in wild, unbridled growth, while disregarding lesser matters. The wood is hard but very elastic, so it's no wonder that people have always made useful implements out of it for ploughing the land, as well as spears, lances, bows and arrows.

In mythology the ash symbolizes the power centre of the world and is the bearer of life. It withstands the destructive forces of nature like no other tree and provides strength amidst all catastrophes. Therefore since the earliest times the ash has been revered in a special way.

The ash has an impressive form: harmonious, slender and majestic. It seldom appears in larger groups. It likes to grow in valleys, alongside streams and on riverbanks. It is at home throughout Europe with a height of up to 40 metres (130 feet). The ash makes high demands on its environment — it loves places with moist air and a lot of light. It takes strength from other plants

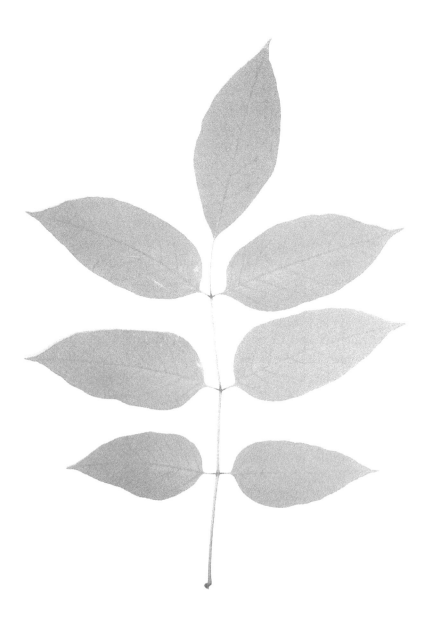

Ash-tree leaf (Fraxinus excelsior)

because it soaks up the water in the ground, so other plants cannot thrive in its vicinity. With its very special properties the ash became symbolic for an ideal in which power and delicacy are united.

In herbal medicine the leaves of the ash were formerly used for gout and rheumatism. They were also recommended as a poultice for healing wounds and broken bones, muscles, jaundice and stone formations. The seeds were even supposed to help with heart murmurs, fluid drainage and as an aphrodisiac. Other sources name ash leaves as a helpful remedy for fertility problems, also for bite wounds. The ash can supposedly reduce a fever, enliven tired feet and help to relieve coughing up blood.

Today it is well known that the principal active ingredient in the ash is coumarin, an anticoagulant. Physiologically they affect the muscles and other 'force organs,' including the uterus, which is a very strong muscle.

In homeopathic doses the ash has a good effect on problems within the female abdomen. It is also used homeopathically for cold sores, gout, rheumatism, fever and hemorrhages. Because it has a close connection to the Bach flower 'olive' it is given to people who suffer from severe exhaustion.

The ash person

Ash mistletoe works to its full potential with slender, athletic women who also have masculine characteristics. Ash people are able to bear heavy burdens over long periods of time. They are friendly and equally devoted to family and the rest of the world. They are ready to serve without putting themselves at the centre of things. Ash people are extremely capable of being burdened and flexible at the same time, and have a high capacity for sacrifice. In modern society these people are mostly women who work and look after their family at the same time.

However, the overwork resulting from having both professional and domestic duties (involvement in two task areas) often leads to becoming ill. In particular these women can suffer from diseases of the female genitals (carcinoma in the uterus) as well as breast cancer and muscular forms of rheumatism.

Hormone imbalances and all forms of cancer that involve a lack of strength and/or a quarrel with one's destiny are also prevalent in ash people.

The ash mistletoe is therefore especially suitable to use after an operation, after radiation or chemotherapy, or other surgery; experience has shown that the ash mistletoe raises life energy, it can improve the general state of health or even bring about healing.

Breast cancer with lymph node metastases

A perceptible swelling was detected in the left breast of a 42-year-old female patient. A subsequent ultrasound examination and mammogram confirmed a suspected tumour. The woman had already felt weak and exhausted for several months. She was a lean, light-skinned type with red hair, very sensitive and sympathetic, who sacrificed herself for her job and her family.

The weakness and exhaustion of this woman, her rather athletic, slender build, the double burden of a job and housekeeping, as well as a hormonal imbalance lead me to see an analogy between the patient and the being of the ash.

Mistletoe therapy was started before her operation. In addition the woman was given some anthroposophically oriented plant remedies. At the subsequent operation the left breast was completely removed; it was followed by chemotherapy and radiation. Just two weeks after the operation the patient was in a relatively good condition. She felt less weak and exhausted, but she feared the cancerous tissue had spread.

After the operation she regularly injected herself with the ash mistletoe preparation. While she did not get the usual fever, her body temperature varied between 35.7 and 37.5°C (96 and

99.5°F) during the course of the day. In the time that followed the woman felt very well on the whole; she had a positive outlook on life. To supplement the mistletoe therapy she was treated with hyperthermia therapy, which raised her temperature to 39°C (102°F).

Three years later the woman felt some hardening in her right breast. The medical examination revealed a carcinoma so another operation became necessary. In the weeks before the operation the woman treated herself with compresses of Swedish bitters (a herbal tonic made of several herbs) and horsetail (*equisitum*), and drank a tea which she had made from horsetail and marigold flowers. During her final check-up a few hours before the operation, something totally unexpected had happened: the metastases had completely dissolved and the operation could be cancelled.

The steady increase in independent decision-making by the patient from one month to the next, and her constant activity after metastases were suspected, point to a growing capability of so-called self-regulation, in which one takes one's life in hand once again.

The ash mistletoe is most suitable at the beginning of mistletoe therapy when the patients are exhausted and weakened as a result of an operation or chemotherapy. In thin female patients the ash mistletoe can also be of good use in the further course of recovery. More than with the other mistletoes one finds an effect similar to hormones — so treatment with ash mistletoe is effectively like an anthroposophical hormone therapy for cancer.

The Scots pine

The wood of the Scots pine (*Pinus sylvestris*) is extraordinarily rich in resin, burns very well and people have always liked to use it as a torch. In mythology there are hardly any references to the Scots pine, but there certainly are to its southern European relation, the stone pine (*Pinus pinea*), which was greatly venerated in Greece and Italy. The names of two Middle-Eastern divinities, Dionysus and Attis, are connected with it. Dionysus is the god of the stone pine; he always appears as the personification of wildness, of an irrational life, given over to impulses and intoxication. There human orgies correspond to the rutting of animals — like the swarming out of the male plant seed, pollen, which sometimes wafts through the air in yellow clouds near the pine woods.

In mythology the stone pine is also associated with a second wild divinity: Attis, who fled from the incestuous love of his own mother, then died after castrating himself; Zeus then turned him into a stone pine. This myth clearly refers to the self-mutilations that were practised to some extent over hundreds of years at rituals in honour of the stone pine. In these old myths one also recognizes clear indications of a passion for waste. In Greek mythology, the cones of the stone pine always symbolized growth and fertility. A stone pine was not so pure and simple as it may appear to us today.

However, in Asian countries the pine stands as a symbol for a calm, orderly being and for constancy. In China pines are planted on graves in order to strengthen the souls of the departed, and it's believed that their life history can be read from its bizarre growth patterns.

It was also popular to spice wine with a pine aroma, and young pine cones were put into the wine barrels. Today the Greek *retsina* still tastes of pine resin.

Besides providing excellent wood for construction and fuel, the pine tree also provides turpentine, resin, white and black pitch, tar, charcoal, soot, various essential oils, a substance similar to paraffin for making candles and creosote. The soft inner bark, cambrium, was used in Scandinavia for baking pine bread. Pine needles were cooked in lye and worked into a fibrous material from which soft flannels were produced, especially recommended for people with gout and rheumatism.

In botany six hundred types of conifer (*Coniferophyta*) are known. About every four years in May a massive production of yellow pollen is blown great distances by the wind. The pine can grow to a height of about forty metres. At the beginning it has a conical shape, then later it looks more like an umbrella. It's a very undemanding tree and grows in places where it's too wet for other trees, too dry, too sunny or too cold. One finds pines growing in sand, limestone ground, gravel or peat soil.

In folk medicine the needles of the pine are considered an excellent remedy for lung diseases, above all for tuberculosis. They mitigate persistent coughs and asthmatic complaints and are used to treat catarrh of the trachea, grippe and chronic bronchitis, but also for headache, toothache, boils, hysteria, hypochondria, as well as for cancers of the female genitalia, kidney diseases and muscle wasting. The main active ingredients are the essential oils, which are predominantly used in catarrhal sicknesses of the upper and lower air passages, also externally for rheumatic complaints and nerve pains. Over and above this, successful results in cases of exhaustion, weakness and anxiety have also been reported.

Today pine shoots and pure essential oils are used as a decongestant, as a mild anti-inflammatory and for improving blood circulation.

Pine is recommended for coughs, colds and flu, usually in the form of a syrup, also externally for minor muscle and nerve pains. Turpentine is the balsam or resinous sap of the pine, and of various other conifers. Formerly it was used for rheumatism and gangrene. Hippocrates, the famous Greek physician, used it as a local softening agent for tumours and for a prolapsed rectum.

Besides the medications from the Scots pine, those derived from the mountain pine (*Pinus mugo*) have long been found valuable. This tree is found high up in the mountains where other trees cannot grow due to the extreme climatic conditions.

Pine substances are used as homeopathic medicines to treat bleeding and irritated mucous membranes, burning pain from lung disease, kidney inflammation, infections of the gall bladder and urethra, against chilblains and vertigo. Pine extracts are also effective for treating dull headaches or tinnitus.

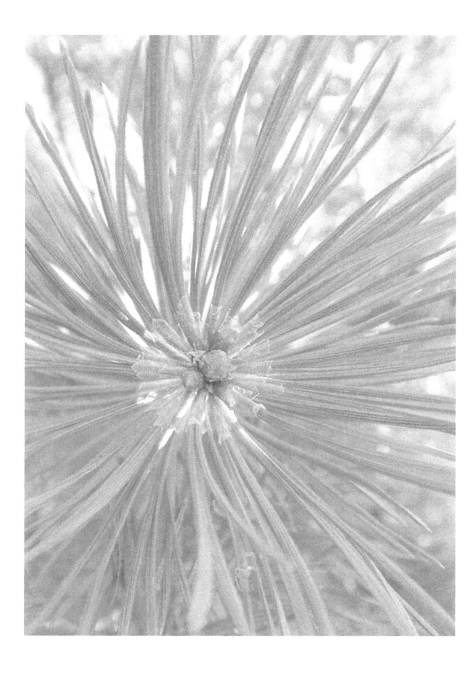

Scots pine-tree needle (Pinus sylvestris)

The pine person

In Bach flower therapy pine is prescribed for people who suffer from self-reproach, guilty feelings and discouragement. They usually set high standards for themselves and feel guilty when they perform no better than anyone else. In their negative mental condition they exhibit an almost masochistic urge for self-sacrifice. Children with pine or stone pine characteristics are often the class scapegoat: they get themselves into situations in which they will be punished. In a positive, transformed condition, pine people have a deep understanding for the faults of others; they accept their own weaknesses and can forgive themselves for their own shortcomings.

Both the Scots and the stone pine are therefore suitable for patients who suffer from severe guilt complexes, self-loathing and who self-harm. The stone-pine mistletoe helps with rheumatic disorders, or when sensitive and generally discontented people suffer from ill health. It is also prescribed for people who are subject to intense passions and drives. (as Dionysus above) but who suppress them and don't want to expose them.

In pine people carcinoma very often appears in the central nervous system, in the female breast, in the skin and the thyroid gland. Pine mistletoe is a remedy for tumours in people who tend to be lean, modest and rather withdrawn from life. Becoming emaciated, especially in the legs, and having a predisposition for respiratory illnesses, are indicative signs.

Thyroid cancer

Nine years ago a forty-year-old woman was found to have a carcinoma in her thyroid gland, which was discovered when she had a goiter removed. She was a very active businesswoman who up to then had never been ill. She assumed the tumour was caused by radiation from Chernobyl. Before she became ill she had occupied herself intensively with the Chernobyl accident and taken care of children who had been injured by the radiation.

For years the patient regularly received injections of pine and ash mistletoe extracts from an anthroposophical doctor. This led to a definite stabilization in her previously unstable condition. However, the development of metastases in the lung could not be prevented, so internal radiation treatments were necessary. Until then her condition had been generally stable; she didn't suffer strongly from anxiety and hadn't lost any weight.

A potentized extract of meadow saffron helped her to endure the regularly performed radiation therapy, and to suppress the resulting nausea that always followed. The last check-up showed her upper neck region to be completely free of carcinomas and the lung metastases were receding. The mistletoe injections are continuing — without them the woman actually feels unwell. In addition she is receiving copper substances in the form of a homeopathically effective remedy for thyroid cancer.

The patient's condition during the nine years of treatment has been good. She is active in sports and has a busy social and professional life as the director of a company.

One can regard the thyroid as the 'brain' of the food assimilation process, which it controls. Apart from making food smaller, breaking it up and decomposing it, this process also destroys the substances that are ingested — hence a kind of 'mutilation,' which takes place in the thyroid carcinoma in a similar way. In this analogy the stone-pine mistletoe helps both against the thyroid cancer as well as the burden of being exposed to radiation. I have supplemented the optimized mistletoe therapy with a copper substance and with the active ingredient of the meadow saffron which mitigates the damage of the radiation treatment.

The lime tree (linden)

The common lime tree has the botanical name *Tilia europaea*. The origin of its name is not clear. It is also called the linden. In the United States 'lime' is used only for the unrelated citrus tree.

The world of legends in every culture is rich in stories about the lime. In Greek mythology Cronus, the father of Zeus, united himself with the nymph Philyra who then gave birth to a divine monster, half-human and half-horse. Frightened and ashamed, Philyra went to her father who managed to turn her into a lime tree.

The famous lovers Philemon and Baucis are also connected to the lime. Philemon turned himself into an oak, Baucis into a lime, which also indicates that in the symbolism of trees the oak represents the masculine principle, the lime the feminine.

The lime tree also plays a central role in the Siegfried legend. When he bathed in the dragon's blood a lime leaf fell between his shoulder blades and afterwards he remained vulnerable in this spot. It was also beneath a lime tree that Hagen delivered the mortal wound. The Song of the Nibelungs is not the only legend in which the lime tree appears; it is the tree of the minnesongs (a form of medieval German love song), altogether a place of love and desire.

The lime tree is also an important tree in settlements. In Central Europe, village life was inconceivable without a lime tree in a central position. For the people it was a place of communication, for the thing (the local assembly), but also for dance performances and festivals.

The common or European lime and the small-leaved lime can be found all over Europe. During blossom time the tree, with up to 60,000 blossoms, is filled with swarms of bees. The wood of the lime tree has a silky sheen, is light and soft, but not very elastic and therefore difficult to work with. It is primarily used for carving. Lime trees grow up to 35 metres in height. While its upward growth stops after 150–180 years, it can then still grow thicker. Lime trees often have an impressive diameter of up to three metres. Limes have become a rarity in forests, because their

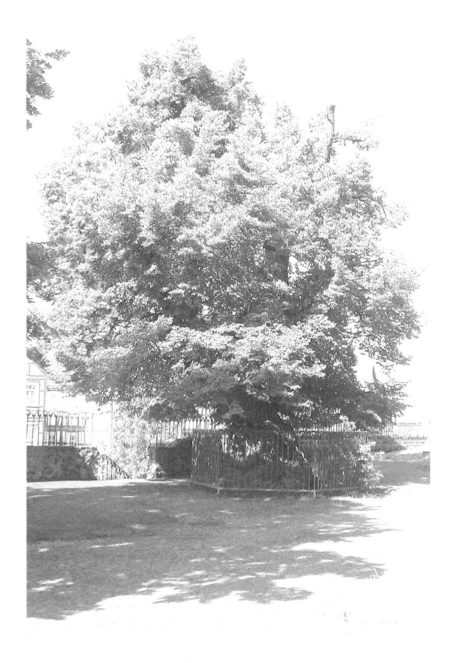

Lime or linden tree (Tilia europea)

soft wood is neither suitable for fuel nor lumber. Linden bast used to be in great demand because sleeping mats and even clothes were made from it.

In terms of medical applications, lime bark was formerly used to treat leprosy, the leaves were used for tumours around the mouth, and the roots and sap against loss of hair.

In the last few centuries, especially through the recommendations of Sebastian Kneipp, lime-blossom tea gained almost legendary importance as an excellent remedy for typical winter ailments like coughs and colds, but also for abdominal complaints.

According to Hildegard of Bingen, lime leaves were good for keeping the eyes clean and could be lain over the eyes and the face. To this day people make compresses from lime-blossom tea and place them on the eyes when they are tired or inflamed. Lime blossom is also good for dizziness and gout conditions.

In folk medicine lime charcoal is taken as a powder. It is an effective disinfectant, it helps with heartburn, with a sensitive digestive system as well as flatulence. Made into a tooth powder, lime charcoal cleans, disinfects and strengthens the gums.

In homeopathy it's considered a valuable remedy for muscular weakness of the eyes, diseases of the jawbone as well as headaches. Lime substances are also used for disorders of the female sexual organs: to strengthen the womb, to treat superficial wounds and swellings of the vulva, inflammation of the pelvis or pains in the womb.

Lime-blossom essences can also help to relieve emotional distress. They promote an atmosphere of warmth and openness, reduce tension and help to strengthen relationships. Lime-flower essence has also proved to be a good medication for people who, as a result of painful experiences, have difficulties in giving and receiving love and affection.

The lime person

Everything about the lime is soft, sweet and gentle. In the lime you can plainly see the maternal principle. Its substances are especially suitable for soft, gentle natures, and above all for women who are a bit plump and very kind of heart. Vulnerable organs are the womb, the female breast, the heart and the lung (which was where Siegfried was mortally wounded) and the eyes. Indications of an inner relationship to the lime are a gentle disposition, but also a strong tendency to perspire. Patients who perspire at night (and more likely those with well-rounded proportions) and who have difficulties in maintaining harmonious family relationships may also have a connection to the lime. In medical literature the lime is even called the 'family therapist' because it helps to resolve social troubles, especially for women who take family conflicts too much to heart and struggle to free themselves from family problem. In those cases the lime is a suitable mistletoe therapy.

Mild depression, with frequent weeping, can sometimes occur in lime people, along with feelings of helplessness and being lost; on the other hand, they are also very grateful for any sympathy and help given.

Lime people are especially liable to develop kidney and lung tumours as well as carcinomas in the bladder and the uterus. Lime types often complain of sharp, stabbing pains in various parts of the body and sometimes feel as if splinters are sticking into the breastbone and the hands and toes. They often like to smoke.

Kidney and lung carcinomas

A seventy-year-old woman had noticed blood in her urine. During the clinical examination a carcinoma was found in the left kidney and also a lung tumour. When the patient's chest cavity was opened a widely extended carcinoma was discovered and the operation was discontinued. The patient had a radiant child-like disposition but had been entirely dependent on others her whole life. She lived with her sister and brother-in-law, who resented her presence, so that there was continual family conflict.

The woman was treated with an optimized lime mistletoe therapy, and recovered rapidly. She continued to ride her bicycle, visited acquaintances and helped with the housework. One evening she asked for a pastor, but as she was doing well he didn't come straightaway. The woman sat before the house in the evening sun and sang some songs with her sister, she said her prayers and then went to bed. The next morning she was found dead.

While the lime mistletoe could not heal the two carcinomas, which were in an advanced stage of development, it probably contributed to an excellent quality of life until the very end. This case illustrates a typical nature with which the lime mistletoe relates: a good-natured but very dependent woman who lived in disturbed family surroundings and had fallen ill.

Stomach tumour

A 65-year-old woman, gentle and corpulent, suffered from a stomach tumour, which was operated on. At home a few years later she fell off her chair and bruised her back and the back of her head. Ever since her fall she felt weak and tired, had back pains and in a short time lost 4 kg (9 lb).

When she came to our clinic she seemed extremely desperate and unhappy. A substantial cause of much of her trouble was due to the constant use of nicotine and alcohol by her husband. This man had always been rejected by the patient's children, so there was continual conflict within the family.

The very gentle, motherly type, permanently weighed down by family conflict, the effects of second-hand smoke and a weak womb, indicated the use of lime mistletoe.

The woman then received an optimized mistletoe therapy with three injections per week in the clinic. Under this treatment she gained 4 kg (9 lb) in weight, fitted in well with the daily routine of the clinic, and was grateful for every therapy and consultation. The difficult family situation was thoroughly discussed. She couldn't decide to take any concrete steps (separation) but she became calmer from day to day and the previous tendency towards depression gradually abated.

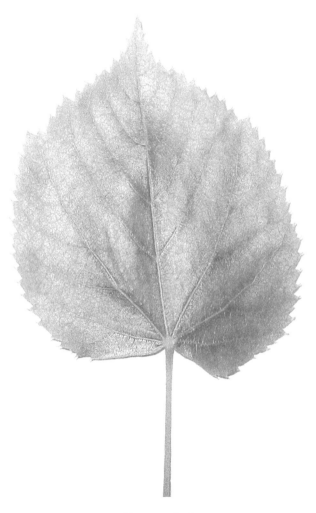

Lime-tree leaf

The almond tree

The almond tree, so people say, is the plant of lovers, entwined with some rather sad stories about the virginal grace of the early blossoms and their tenderness, because they often wither away in a spring frost. The almond has appeared throughout Middle-Eastern and Greek culture as far back as the Stone Age. It is supposed that the almond — also often mentioned in the Bible — is the oldest cultivated fruit in the world. The seven-branched Jewish menorah is an imitation of the almond tree. In 812 the Emperor Charlemagne ordered the almond tree to be introduced into the royal farmlands. In the Middle Ages almonds were highly valued, and in the fourteenth century almonds were one of the main goods traded internationally. Sweet almonds are used in the production of marzipan.

The almond, like the apple and pear and most other fruit trees, belongs to the rose family. But the difference with the almond is that we eat the seed instead of the flesh of the fruit; however, this seed is not a nut, from a botanical point of view.

The almond tree thrives best in mountainous regions with hot, dry summers and cool winters. The bush or small tree has straight, bare branches, which are thorny in the wild variety and have grey bark. The almond shell is quite flat, wedge-shaped with furrowed wrinkles. The cinnamon-brown seed it contains is also flat and about two centimetres long. Depending on the variety it can be very bitter. The bitter almond contains a glycoside that breaks down into prussic acid, and can be fatally poisonous.

The almond oil extracted from the kernel has been used since antiquity for skin inflammations because of its softening and moistening effects. Poultices were made from the skin or root of the bitter almond and used to clean the face; they were also effective against eczema and other skin ailments, and relieved headaches when placed over the temples. The bitter almond was also believed to be effective for diseases of the lung, liver and kidneys. In the Middle Ages an aqueous solution containing bitter almond was prescribed for coughs, as an emetic and for nausea.

Today this solution is used as a component in lotions and salves, above all in the treatment rheumatism. But because of the poisonous nature of the bitter almond, it's important not to self-medicate! This bitter-almond solution is also used when someone complains of severe pains in the tonsils, when the throat and gums are enflamed and to treat severe coughs which lead to chest pains. An overdose may give rise to the typical symptoms of cyanide poisoning — dizziness, stammering, convulsive laughter, facial spasms and finally loss of consciousness. In homeopathic doses the almond is effective in treating heart and lung illnesses that cause breathing difficulties, because like many rose plants it contains hydrogen cyanide. Almond oil is used as a basic ingredient in cosmetic and medicinal skin ointments. There is no further known use of the almond in medical practice.

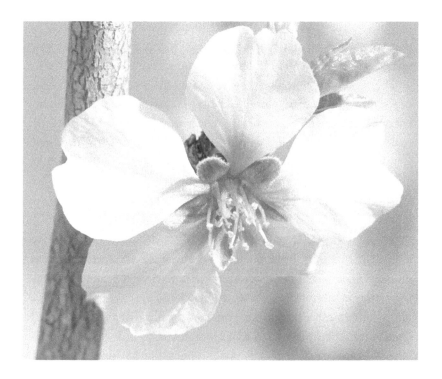

Almond-tree blossom (Prunus amygdalus)

The almond-tree person

Almond people carry the mark of the tree in themselves to an astonishing degree. On the outside they appear to be gentle, soft, compliant and peaceful characters, who usually express their emotions with difficulty or not at all. Frequently one suspects that these patients were psychologically injured by their parents or by their social environment, even to the point of being abused. They are vulnerable and try to compensate for the 'social pain' they have suffered by over-achieving. Some of them show signs of inner embitterment and one is struck by their inability or unwillingness to speak about past injustices. But outwardly they still show a friendly, lovable disposition.

Physically they are primarily at risk from diseases of the neck area and lungs. Asthmatics are particularly at risk, as well as those who haven't overcome grief from a previous relationship, who prefer to hide their emotions and withdraw into their own bitterness. Carcinomas frequently develop in the lymphatic system and as malignant tumours in the skin. According to current experience, the active ingredients of the almond mistletoe are now used almost specifically to treat skin diseases and often effect a cure within a few weeks.

Skin cancer

Thirteen years ago a 53-year-old woman was diagnosed with skin cancer; since then a lymph node metastasis appeared on her neck and, from the CT scan, a brain metastasis was suspected. The dermatology clinic recommended chemotherapy, which the woman declined.

During the examination to determine the optimized mistletoe treatment, the patient also reported a lymph node swelling in the neck that she had noticed six months earlier. When under stress her hearing was poor and she smoked ten cigarettes per day. She said she was basically a happy person, but reserved. She had no happy relationships: her father died when she was nine years old; at the age of seventeen her only daughter was born. She always subordinated herself to her husband, who had died of a pancreatic tumour some years earlier.

The location of the tumour and the soul type of the patient — a gentle, perfectionist kind of person, who had absorbed a lot of grief and was embittered and disappointed by life, yet appeared obliging on the outside — all this indicated the almond mistletoe. Also her prior history with its numerous psychological shocks was typical, according to my experience, of an almond-mistletoe patient.

Therefore therapy with almond mistletoe was prescribed in addition to homeopathic doses of bromine. Fortunately, half a year later, no evidence of a brain metastasis could be found. The woman no longer felt weak, she could sleep well again and had become much calmer, which she said her friends had noticed. She had put aside her previous hectic ways and her general condition was stable. The lymph-node swelling had disappeared.

The almond mistletoe treatment is being pursued at changing potency levels.

Skin cancer with metastases

A 57-year-old patient had lived with a virolous abscess on his left eye for seventeen years. During an examination metastases were found at the head of the pancreas and the right lobe of the liver. These two carcinomas had already been discovered respectively five and two years previously.

The latest examination also raised the suspicion of further metastases in the neck and shoulder. After the surgical removal of the abdominal metastases half a year before, the patient had lost 10 kg (22 lb) — he now weighed 63 kg (139 lb) — but his weight remained steady. He appeared to be gentle and stable; he had enough strength to take care of himself.

He had suffered from indigestion and mild stomach pains for several years. During his school days he had difficulty emptying his bowels and suffered from a bloated abdomen. The man had always swallowed down his anger without defending himself. In his professional and private lives he embodied the ideal of the 'silent' perfectionist. His first marriage had ended unhappily, but he was now happily married again. According to his wife, he needed to feel safe and secure in the world around him.

During our conversation the man reported that he often felt sick after breakfast, which he blamed on his sensitivity to the smell of certain foods. When he felt sick he also complained about ice-cold feet, but at the same time he would be on the verge of perspiring (dumping syndrome). He could eat quite a lot, but had no great appetite. His digestion was normal, his stools rather light in colour, and since the operation he often suffered from flatulence. He slept through the night and only seldom had dreams.

He appears as a very gentle, perfectionist sort of person who swallows a lot of grief and at the same time is outwardly friendly and obliging. This psychological profile and the location of the tumour were for me a clear analogy of the character of the almond tree. Therefore I prescribed an almond-mistletoe therapy for the patient. This was supplemented by injections of a silver preparation twice a week.

With optimized mistletoe therapy the man regained strength within a few weeks, could carry heavy sacks and do without lunch breaks. Despite any concerns for the future he built a house.

His body weight remained stable at 64 kg (141 lb). He often had a ravenous appetite and could eat excessively. His indigestion was better, he had regular bowel movements, he no longer suffered from nausea or stomach pains, his feet were warm and he didn't perspire. The mistletoe injections were followed by the desired strong reactions with painful swellings for one to three days.

This case study and the man's biography are typical of the curative possibilities of an optimized almond-mistletoe therapy. The previous history of almond-mistletoe patients almost always shows severe social distress and blows of fate. People who suffer such burdens are gentle as a rule, but introverted and even embittered. More than any other carcinoma, skin cancers (malignant melanoma and basal cell carcinoma) seem to respond to almond mistletoe, and after the injections there are almost always severe initial reactions with fever or strong inflammation at the site of the injection.

The poplar

The name of one species of poplar, the aspen (*Populus tremula*) presumably comes from the constant movement of its rustling leaves. Everyone in Germany is familiar with the saying, 'to tremble like an aspen leaf.' In France the poplar is, next to the oak, the freedom tree, the 'tree of the people.' In the word *peuplier* (poplar) we find the concept of *peuple*.

In Greek mythology poplars have a connection with the underworld and with prophecy. In this regard the white poplar symbolizes peaceful death, in contrast with the black poplar, which is actually feared as a bringer of misfortune. This gloomy aspect was also represented on the Field of Mars in Rome, where the funeral pyre for the cremation of the emperors was surrounded by black poplars. Another story describes the creation of the poplar from the Heliades, the daughters of the sun god Helios. They were overcome with grief for the loss of their brother, Phaeton, who had been hurled down from the heavens, so Zeus turned them into poplar trees.

Poplars are among the fastest growing native timber trees. They are divided into many kinds: the white poplar, the black poplar and the aspen. The aspen likes light and makes no special demands on the environment. Poplars can grow to a height of 10–30 metres (30–100 feet). They grow with positively breathtaking speed; to grow them you need only stick a branch in the earth, and little rootlets begin to develop right away. Pointed or pyramid shaped poplars are like oversized index fingers which reach up towards the sky. Like an army of gigantic soldiers they line the edges of avenues and rivers. Napoleon had them planted along his military highways as an unmistakable expression of his claim to their possession.

Poplars much prefer to grow by the water. They are pioneer plants that settle in desert lands. With their roots they firm up the edges of streams, swamps and rivers. The leaves are light on one side, dark on the other — a play of change, like yin and yang, like sun and moon.

Poplar wood is used above all to make cellulose and for kindling. It's light, soft, light-coloured and easy to split. Matches are made from poplar wood. It's not very hard or durable since it grows so fast. Its bark is used for tanning, its twigs and branches for making traps, and the buds and leaves were formerly symbolically worn to attract money and to become wealthy.

Poplars are used in medicine over Europe, America and China. The Native Americans used it as a remedy for coughing, the buds of the black poplar were used for haemorrhoids and burn wounds. In China poplar ingredients provided remedies for hip pains and incontinence and the buds were used for burns and inflammations. In Europe poplar extracts have been used to remedy diarrhoea, gonorrhoea and leucorrhoea, for heart burn, bladder inflammations and chronically excessive menstrual flow. The leaves were recommended for incontinence in the elderly. The aspen was also believed to help with swellings of the prostate. In Russia the white poplar (*Populus alba*) was successfully used to treat malaria. In phytotherapy the leaves of the bud and the bark are used as a bitter tonic to help with digestive and liver complaints. The aspen contains salicylic acid, which gives it an effect similar to aspirin. This also explains its use for malaria. It's a good remedy when there is pain from inflamed joints. There are also reports of success in cases of weakness of the uterine muscles.

In homeopathy the poplar is used to treat bladder problems in older people, as well as for heartburn and for enlargement of the prostate.

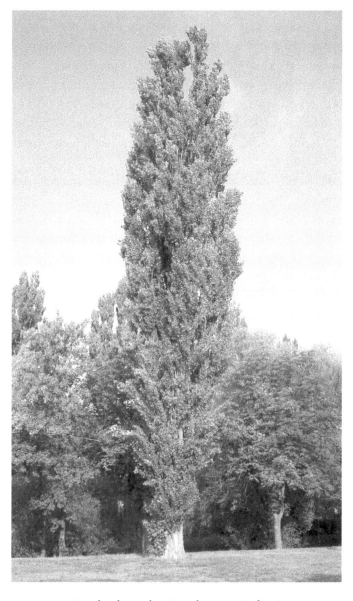

Lombardy poplar (Populas nigra 'italica')

The poplar person

Poplar substances are particularly suited to tall people who have a tendency for obedience — almost like that of a soldier. Patients who are driven very strongly — often without any cause — by anxiety or unconscious tensions are typical poplar people, above all when they stand on the threshold of death. These people actually tremble like aspen leaves and they often let themselves be influenced by superstitious ideas and presentiments. They occupy themselves intensively with death and religion and with imagined misfortunes that may be about to happen.

When poplar people get sick with cancer, they suffer in particular from these indefinable fears. They are afraid something awful could happen at any moment, are overly nervous and have a constant need to talk.

With these patients carcinomas usually grow very fast. Metastases are often already found at the first diagnosis. Poplar preparations seem to work well for carcinomas that produce night sweating and severe exhaustion, as well as for tumours that cause severe pain. They are especially good for bladder cancer and carcinomas of the prostate.

The poplar mistletoe is presumed to be one of the safest mistletoes to use for causing a fever (its use for malaria tertiana) and therefore, not unjustly, is popular and listed by many producers of mistletoe preparations.

Prostate cancer and bone metastases

A lean and weakened eighty-year-old patient with a prostate carcinoma and bone metastases in the dorsal and sacral vertebrae and in the upper thighs and upper arms came to the clinic after surgical removal of the prostate and after repeated hormone treatments. The patient had a constant need to talk; he was afraid of the consequences of his illness. He couldn't accept the short life-expectancy that had previously been predicted for him; he still wanted to have a good life for a few years. The bald-headed patient was by nature a merry Rhinelander. He felt chilly a lot and he had to get up several times a night to go to the toilet.

The patient's extreme weakness and exhaustion originally gave me an indication towards the ash. Although the location of the tumour, the man's constant fear of a spread of the disease and his continual fear-filled talk and 'babbling' pointed to the poplar.

The patient was first treated with a preparation of ash mistletoe, but there was no substantial improvement in his general condition.

The character of the illness, the rapid growth of the metastases and the continued presence of the patient's fears then caused me to switch the therapy to the poplar mistletoe.

In the following three weeks the patient had a feverish ague and temperatures reaching 40°C (104°F); then, beside the fall of the patient's excessively high blood pressure, the tumour marker levels also fell from one hundred to almost zero within three months. The average body temperature was 37°C (99.5°F) (before it had been 35.9°C/ 96.5°F).

Three years after therapy was begun, the general condition of the patient is still good, and the numerous metastases in the skeletal system have somewhat receded. However the man still reports of sleeplessness, although he can do without alcohol. During the three years of treatment in which he was treated regularly with mistletoe and silver substances he did not lose any weight. His fears have largely vanished and he feels well in his body. He has already reached his aim to enjoy life for a few more years.

The fir

The fir tree (*Abies*) has for centuries been inseparably connected with the Christmas festival. It's believed that the first Christmas tree stood in Strasbourg cathedral in 1538, and since around 1870 the custom became widespread throughout Europe. The decoration of fir trees with apples and nuts symbolizes the miracle of Christ's birth. The fir tree is the tree of life in winter, a symbol of the transformation of hard ice into life and of death's night into the light of the world — hence also Christmas candles. The fir as Christmas tree has become a myth, and it has a particularly deep spiritual relationship with the mistletoe.

In German society the fir's place was taken by the spruce so it doesn't feature prominently in our culture. Firs reach a maximum age of 180–200 years, with a height of 30–40 metres (100–130 feet) and a diameter of one metre. An older tree has a long tap root and a flattened crown that looks like a stork's nest. However, when the tree is dying these crowns take on a broom-like shape.

The wood is light in colour and in weight, it's easily split and the bark has a reddish shimmer. The seed and its covering are not sharply differentiated. The wood dries rapidly and tears easily. The needles all drop off every six to eleven years. Firs only begin to bloom when they are about thirty years old. They prefer shady places with deep, fresh, moist, fruitful soil and with loam going into clay. The fir cannot stand acid soils, as was discovered when their forests started to die out some time ago.

Fir is a preferred wood for making sounding boards in musical instruments; other uses include the production of furniture, wooden containers, matches and shingles. In earlier times it was the most important wood in ship building.

The resin of the fir was formerly used for healing purposes; it was also traded as Strasbourg turpentine. The resin smells of lemon or spices. It's a component of salves for rheumatism and arthritis and is supposed to be able to firm up the gums. Fresh fir sprouts

— just like pine branches — are used to treat coughs and colds, as well as weak lungs and bronchitis: these are recommendations of Sebastian Kneipp. For the mystic Hildegard of Bingen, the fir was a symbol of strength. According to her, ghosts hate the wood of the fir and avoid places where it grows.

In homeopathy substances are used from only two types of fir, commonly known as black spruce (*Abies nigra*) and hemlock spruce (*Abies Canadensis*), which have a connection with the mucous membranes of the stomach. The symptoms that call for the use of fir mistletoe can be diverse, but fir preparations are almost always appropriate when the patient feels a 'wintry cold'

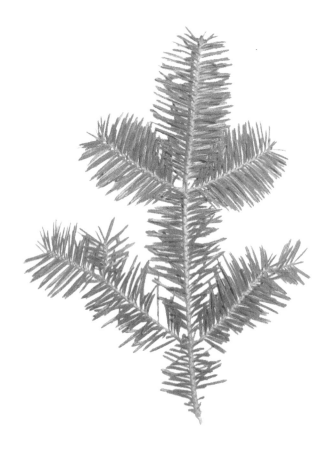

Balsam-fir branch (abries balsamea)

within himself. Homeopathy recommends fir as a remedy for patients who suffer from a constant appetite, with a gnawing feeling of hunger in the upper abdomen; who feel as if their blood is running through them like ice water; who suffer from stomach pains after eating, and digestive complaints in elderly people.

The fir person

Fir mistletoe is appropriate for patients who have a strong feeling of responsibility and who prefer to remain remote from events and from other people. They are often described as stubborn and inflexible because of this attitude. At the same time such people have an entirely clear conception of how others, as well as they themselves, need to behave in particular situations.

In fir people carcinomas of the lung, the aesophagus, the stomach and the intestines occur especially frequently, in men also in the prostate. Metastases in the spinal column have also been observed remarkably often.

Patients who can be helped by fir mistletoe often feel the cold very strongly, and particularly notice this cold feeling in the blood, the stomach or the lungs. Fir mistletoe also strengthens the lung tissue, so it's used to treat chronic bronchitis.

Prostate cancer

A sixty-year-old patient had his prostate surgically removed. He was tall and lean, and besides cancer of the prostate he had carcinomas in the lymph nodes that were already advanced. Afterwards he had hormone therapy and radiation, but these had to be discontinued after a short time because of further complaints. Since the operation the man complained of incontinence, especially in the afternoon.

During the consultation it turned out that the patient had suffered from constipation since childhood with at most one bowel movement each week. He always had cold hands and furthermore he often had no sensation in his fingers.

The man seldom had dreams, was very nervous and felt that he could no longer manage his work. During the medical consultation he was reserved and quiet. His life basically revolved around home and sports. His life was determined by rather rigid moral principles.

On the basis of the 'hard morality' of the man, because of his principles and his happiness with hearth and home, the oak mistletoe seemed to be appropriate for him. Therefore, I initially prescribed an optimized oak-mistletoe therapy for the patient, supplemented by a homeopathic aluminum preparation. Just a month after the injection, the man could sleep better, the constipation had gone and his bowel movements had normalized.

Over the course of time, however, he complained of an increasing feeling of cold in his arms and legs, a varicose vein in his hip became inflamed and he had severe pressure and other difficulties with his stomach.

The constant feeling of cold and the considerable pressure on his stomach indicated the fir mistletoe for a man of his lean build. I also saw an analogy to the fir in his relatively rigid moral stance.

On the basis of the new situation, his therapy was changed from oak to fir mistletoe, and the patient now received silver instead of aluminum as a metal containing substance. Hyperthermia therapy was also given. These combined therapies produced a good increase in weight and the man felt very well — shamefully well, as he himself put it. The CT scan, however, showed a small source in the lung, and it was suspected that metastases might occur.

As a result the mistletoe treatment was continued, and five years after the critical consultation no lung metastases have been confirmed. The tumour marker levels had decreased and at the final examination were no longer in evidence. The man no longer acted so frigidly in his relationships with other people, but had 'thawed.' He was, however, not yet entirely cured of his incontinence.

The elm

The Romans called the elm *Ulmus*. The wych elm or Scots elm (*Ulmus gabra*) derives its name from the old Germanic root word *Wice*, from which we get the English word 'witch.'

In Greek mythology the elm was above all the symbol for grief, and was therefore planted in groves where the dead were buried. In Germanic mythology, man grew out of the elm. Just as the ash represented the ancestral mother, so the elm embodied the ancestral father of the human race. It is also the tree of St Martin: it was believed that an elm grew up from his pilgrim staff. Elms often stand before churches named after a martyr. This may be connected to a Greek tradition, but perhaps also because elms 'bleed.'

The elm is America's tree of freedom, the 'tree of liberty,' because on August 19, 1765 two straw dolls, which represented British colonial power, were hung up on the old elm tree by the frog pond in Boston; this marked the beginning of the War of Independence. After the victory a joyful festival was held at the same spot in May 1786.

The elm is also found all over Europe and Asia. It grows rapidly in its youth and generally reaches a height of almost forty metres (130 feet) after thirty years. The crown is high, roundly vaulted and amply branched. Elms show a need for warmth. The root system is well developed, the bark is a grey-brown with long deep furrows and is rich in cork. The asymmetry of the leaves is striking. Together with the hazel and the willow the elm opens its blossoms in the spring.

The elm loves sunny hills, copses and meadows; it's one of the trees most in need of warmth and prefers fresh soil rich in nutrients. It's a tough wood, however it tears easily, but is hard to

split. Wheel hubs and spokes, tubs, waterwheels and well troughs
are made from elm — symbolizing movement and transformation.
Furniture and inlaid floors are made out of the heart-wood with
its lively grain. Woodcarvers and sculptors like to use elm wood
because of its maleable structure. Rudolf Steiner created his
famous sculpture, The Representative of Man, out of elm wood. In
this work the hardening and volatizing forces of the human being
are shown in a well-balanced way.

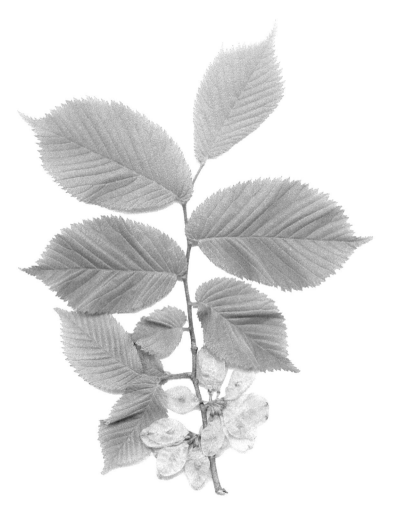

Elm-tree foliage and seeds (Ulmus)

The elm has become a tree of the city; it can cope well with polluted air. However, unfortunately today about ninety per cent of elms suffer from a disease (Dutch elm disease) caused by an insect and a fungus. They destroy the inner passages of the tree and cut it off from its source of life. First the leaves wither, then the branches dry out.

The active substances of the elm were always regarded as having healing properties for the skin and for wounds. Hildegard of Bingen recommended the elm as a remedy for gout: whoever bathes in water heated with elm wood is freed from malice and filled with 'happiness and good thoughts.' In folk medicine elm is used to treat diarrhoea, chronic skin rashes, gout and rheumatism, for haemorrhages and fever, abscesses and boils. An elm wash is supposed to hasten scar formation; for rheumatism the bark and leaves are both used. The principal ingredients are tanning and mucilage, potassium and bitter substances.

In homeopathy, medicinal substances from the elm are used to treat deafness and itchy legs, but also for rheumatic ailments and for muscle and ligament pains.

The elm person

As a rule elm patients are tough diligent people who do good work, are glad to help others, don't go to extremes, and remarkably often follow their inner calling in life. They are honest towards themselves and other people.

However, they sometimes feel overworked, which can lead to depression and lack of courage. Then even those of strong character struggle to see beyond the current problem or find a solution. In such situations they often judge themselves to be weak, overburdened and worn out. The active substances in elm can help in such seemingly insoluble situations; they can help people to view conflict from another perspective and to loosen the worsening situation. Change and transformation are typical strengths of elm people.

But they are often not sufficiently awake to themselves when harm threatens them; they are often in danger of becoming sick from negative influences in the environment of our time. The character of the elm tree, which has a special position among mistletoe trees, explains this: no tree is so open to the environment as the elm, and no other tree is so much like the human being of our Aquarian age, who is open and willing to change. The elm is also like modern man in his weakness to become asymmetrical (one-sided) and to succumb to life's temptations.

In elm people carcinomas typically occur in the organ most open to the outside world — the lungs. And because the elm reacts so sensitively to poisons in the environment, there's an analogy to that group of patients who very frequently become sick with lung tumours, i.e. those who smoke.

Lung cancer with lymph node metastases

A CT scan revealed a 3.5 cm (1 ½ in) tumour in the left lung of a 67-year-old patient, which had encroached on to the adjacent arterial branches, with metastases in the lymph vessels. His left vocal cord was also damaged so he could only speak with a hoarse voice. Because the illness was so far advanced, neither radiation nor chemotherapy was advisable. The lung tumour was surgically removed. Its origin was apparently due to nicotine abuse — the man had smoked twenty cigarettes a day for fifty years. As a child he had been ill with pleurisy and inflammation of the lungs.

The lung cancer of this patient was clearly caused by the continual self-inflicted damage of smoking; with men this circumstance alone points to the elm. However, in the case of corpulent and soft-hearted women of a gentle nature, there would in such cases be more of an analogy to the lime. The lung itself is asymmetrically formed, just like the elm leaf (two lung lobes on the left, three on the right) and is known to be the inner human organ most open to the environment.

After the operation the patient was treated with elm-mistletoe therapy and a homeopathic medicine from the tobacco plant.

Despite the advanced cancer, the patient made rapid progress in his therapy and the accompanying dose of cortisone could be reduced. The damaged vocal cord was also getting better. Within three weeks the patient gained 2 kg (4 1/2 lb). A year later, the man developed acute shortness of breath and pneumonia. The investigative CT scan produced an unexpected result: there was nothing striking of any kind, no metastases.

During the next four years the formerly seriously ill patient lived without any problems. The treatment consisted solely in the continuation of the elm-mistletoe therapy. He even improved his condition by running for up to 6 km (3 3/4 miles). Five years after the almost hopeless first diagnosis the man died from a stroke, which had no connection with the original cancer.

The willow

The Latin name for willow is *Salix* and is derived from the Indo-European root *selk* (to wind, to turn). In German it is also popularly called a 'head willow': if the young trunk is polled at a man's height and the sprouts are cut off every second or third winter, then a head is formed. The willow is also called 'pussy willow' and in some parts of Britain and Europe is still know as 'palm.' In many parts of Europe the willow was used as a substitute for palms when decorating churches on Palm Sunday.

In Greek mythology the willow was consecrated to Artemis, the mother goddess, and to Demeter, the goddess of fertility. She was the symbol for the unbounded life forces — she ruled over the ploughlands and fields, the meadows, rivers and streams. However, besides poplars willows were also regarded as trees of the underworld. In the Middle Ages they were even known as witch trees: witches' brooms were supposedly braided out of willow switches.

There are about 250 types of willow throughout the world. For curative purposes silver and black willows are mostly used. Willows grow rapidly; even small willow shoots quickly put out roots. They develop into a tree 20–25 metres high and become hollow in later years. The short trunk soon puts out branches and carries an irregularly formed, loose crown. From April onwards, 3–6 cm-long (1–2 in) catkins develop.

Willows like to grow in fresh, moist, deep soil and need a lot of light. They love flowing water and are often found beside rivers, watery meadows, ponds and lakes. Old willows have an ochre-grey bark with furrows and rib-like markings. Young trees, on the other hand, have a smooth grey-white bark. The most prominent member of the willow family — the weeping willow — has impressive drooping branches. Willows produce

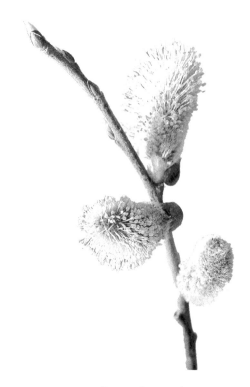

Pussy-willow catkins (Salix caprea)

a lot of pollen and are therefore loved by bees, especially in the spring. Cuttings for new shoots are often taken from willows; the flexibility and perpetual youth of the willow is demonstrated by the ability to braid its young branches and because they are quickly and easily regenerated — you only have to poke them into a moist soil.

The willow was strikingly described by Annette von Droste-Huelshoff. In her novelette *Ledwina* she wrote:

> The willows, for example, have something touching for me.
> They show a peculiar confusion of nature: the branches
> are coloured, the leaves grey — they appear like pretty but
> sickly children whose hair one night turned white from
> fright.

The willow's wood is soft with coarse fibres and is easily bendable; it dries quickly and can be easily worked. It is used for boxes, baskets, clogs, wood shavings, in boat construction, safety matches and in the paper industry. The branches are used for basket-making.

In traditional European medicine the willow was preferentially used for rheumatic and flu-like infections — namely for complaints that are worsened by dampness. This is indicated by the plant's characteristics and its close proximity to water. It has proved itself in healing muscular pain and in its use to promote urination and treat circulatory ailments. Based on its ability in reducing fever, willow was formerly used to treat malaria, as well as for strong menstrual bleeding and the treatment of cuts.

Today willow bark is also to treat head colds and as an enlivening tonic to promote regeneration. But the main use is for circulation problems. The black willow is believed to have a normalizing effect on sexual activity — sometimes stimulating, sometimes calming. It is said to help with constipation and pains in the ovaries and uterus.

In homeopathy the black willow's substances work favourably on the sexual organs of both sexes. It moderates sexual passions and over-excitability. Pain in the testicles and ovaries, as well as ailments of the menstrual cycle, are treated with willow extracts. Preparations from the silver willow help to loosen up patients with rigid behavioural patterns, to make them more flexible and enable them to conduct their life with confidence once again.

The willow person

The willow and its mistletoe have an analogy with patients who are lacking in life forces. This is usually the case following chemotherapy when people's bodies are weakened. The willow helps with all those ailments that need 'regeneration.' This applies particularly to patients who have become stultified in their thinking and spiritual life. The healing power of the willow became world famous with aspirin; this active substance regulates management of the fluids in the human body like hardly any other — and just like the acetic acid of the willow, its mistletoe also promotes circulation. It makes both body and spirit flexible again and helps to lift inward-looking people out of their social backwater.

Willow people often tend to bear grudges and feel bitter. With this negative attitude, they then blame other people for their own misfortunes. They envy others who are doing well, but otherwise show little interest in them — with the result that they often isolate themselves and, inwardly disappointed, they withdraw from social life. The willow mistletoe can help such patients to recover their positive attitude: taking control of their lives and becoming architects of their own destiny, instead of being its victims.

Heraclitus' axiom, 'Everything flows,' can be applied to the willow in a special way: in the human being it promotes the capacity to convert one's ideas and aims into deeds, and even to transform conflicts and problems into living energy. Thus the willow helps those people who have become a shadow of their self to find a way out of the nether world and back into real life.

In cancer therapy willow mistletoe has proven itself above all with diseases of the bone marrow, with tumours of the ovaries and testicles, and with rheumatic ailments. Willow mistletoe is especially helpful in treating joint problems. With rheumatism, but even more with fibromyalgia (a painful disease of the muscle connective tissue), willow mistletoe possesses the greatest healing power of all mistletoes.

Leukaemia

The patient had suffered from leukaemia for twelve years. Before that he was never seriously ill, but as child he had diphtheria. His wife had committed suicide 25 years ago. His leukaemia was treated with chemotherapy and several blood transfusions. This led to pneumonia, which was treated with antibiotics that lowered the fever and reduced the inflammation. With a fluid-reduction therapy, the stoppage in the lungs and the effusion in the pleura also got better. Chemotherapy was discontinued because of the serious inflammation of both lungs, but in time the condition of the blood got worse.

In his desperate state, the man, who was very lean and slightly hunched, sought out our clinic. He grumbled about the clinic for acute cases and its doctors who had 'inflicted' chemotherapy on him. His overall condition was now considerably reduced; he had lost 10 kg (22 lb) in the previous weeks. The great negativity of the patient and his inner hardening, which expressed themselves in the leukaemia as a kind of 'cooling off' of his circulation, made a good match with the character of the willow and its mistletoe.

Therefore the patient was prescribed a willow mistletoe therapy, and in addition he received anthroposophical medicines to stimulate his appetite.

With this treatment the laboratory tests improved significantly, and for the first time in twelve years there was a large reduction of cancer cells in his blood. The man's weight increased by 3 kg

(6 ¹/₂ lb) and when, after four weeks, he could be released from the clinic his general condition was good and he was at peace with himself.

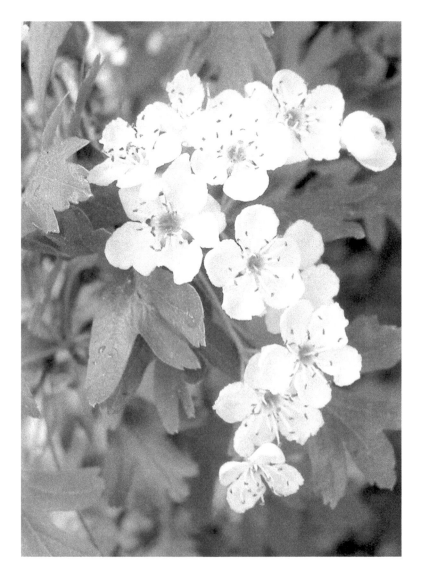

Hawthorn flowers (Crataegus)

The hawthorn

The now disused Latin name *Crataegus oxyacantha* contains the words 'firm' and 'sharp thorns.' The German name of 'white thorn' refers to its white blossoms. Now termed *Crataegus laevigita*, the hawthorn is also known as May. Another name is the 'bread and butter' tree as farmers nibbled the leaves to take the edge off their hunger.

We know from Greek mythology about the drunken feasts that took place to celebrate the coming of new wine. Three days later, so it was said, the souls of the dead appeared to visit the world of the living. Hawthorn branches were picked for protection against them, to ward off mischief. According to Christian tradition, Christ's crown was woven out of hawthorn. In the past, branches of hawthorn, which blossom at Christmas time, were always nailed above the door of the cow barn to drive away evil spirits and protect the cattle from sicknesses. Amulets were also made from hawthorn.

The hawthorn grows as a bush with many branches to a height of two to three metres by the side of fields and roads. People like to use it as a living windbreak. It blossoms from May to June. Striking features of the hawthorn bush are the closely intertwined stems, as well as the thickly crowded, intricate and impenetrable branch systems. On the other hand, a blossoming hawthorn bush gives the impression of an impulsive outburst of strength. The putrid fish-like odour of the blossoms, however, is rather unpleasant. The hard and very tough wood was formerly used for lathe work, but also for walking sticks, tool handles and threshing flails.

In medical science the hawthorn has only been used since the Middle Ages. In the middle of the nineteenth century an Irish doctor achieved great results by treating numerous heart ailments with hawthorn. In Lorraine, France, the hawthorn was reputed to be a well-known remedy for heart palpitations and sleeplessness. Its fruit was recognized as a very effective remedy for side stitches, colic and diarrhoea, kidney stones, dysentery and excessively heavy menstruation.

To this day, tea made from hawthorn blossoms is highly recommended in folk medicine for treating elderly patients with heart problems and for lowering high blood pressure in cases of arteriosclerosis. Hawthorn preparations are also beneficial because they do not contain harmful poisons. Hawthorn extracts calm the nervous system and strengthen the heart and circulation in older people.

Today the main indications for the use of hawthorn are: heart problems, fits of tiredness, states of exhaustion and minor disturbances in heart rhythm. Hawthorn has also proven that it can help to strengthen patients following infectious diseases.

In homeopathy the hawthorn is recognized as a very effective treatment for patients suffering from an irregular heartbeat and sleeplessness, as well as with high blood pressure. Hawthorn substances are said to be able to dissolve arterial deposits. Extreme shortness of breath from the slightest exertion, pain in the heart region and under the left collarbone, as well as a blue-red colouration in the fingers and feet are characteristic symptoms for using hawthorn treatments. Hawthorn also serves well as a soothing medication for patients who are angry and irritable.

The hawthorn person

Mistletoe from the hawthorn has a warming effect. It is above all suitable for people who are unable to express their feelings. Hawthorn blossoms mitigate pain — be it from love, broken hearts, disappointment, anger or bitterness — when the feelings of men, women or children are hurt, when they are lacking in warmth of soul and heartfelt sympathy.

Patients who, besides having impoverished feelings are also stressed by too much work, are beneficially warmed by the hawthorn mistletoe. This is especially important for people whose nose and extremities are discoloured with a reddish blue. Sick people whose masculine aspects (animus) in the Jungian sense are very developed, but who have neglected their feminine side (anima), can also be helped by hawthorn. This is also true for patients who have insufficiently 'nourished' their heart; in the medical literature the hawthorn is sometimes described as 'oatmeal for the heart.'

Tumerous illnesses of the blood occur remarkably often in hawthorn people, such as the various forms of leukaemia. Rheumatic ailments, high blood pressure, as well as heart and circulation problems are typical of hawthorn people.

Leukaemia

Three years ago, a 72-year-old female patient — who had already had two heart attacks and suffered from considerable narrowing of the blood vessels in her legs, head and heart — had become sick with leukaemia, a few months after the death of her husband. She reported that she constantly felt tired and worn out and could hardly venture out of the house any more. She always felt cold; in particular, her fingers and toes never got warm any more.

The woman had worked all her life. Even following the birth of her children, she only allowed herself a short maternity leave. Furthermore, on top of her professional work she was always active in and took leading roles in social institutions such as the Rotary Club.

The widespread narrowing of the blood vessels, the hardening tendency in general, but also her over-emphasis on professional life — this pronounced left-brain performance went hand in hand with her disregard of emotions and her inability to keep warm, especially in her legs. All this indicated a relationship to the hawthorn. Consequently I prescribed a treatment with hawthorn mistletoe for the woman.

Within a few weeks, the previously heightened number of white blood corpuscles (leukocytes) was reduced by one third, a result which had not been attained in the years before. Also the thorough warming of the body, especially the legs, was increased. The patient felt stronger and even hoped to be able to take up her beloved golf again in the spring.

More than the other mistletoes the hawthorn mistletoe appears to suit patients with serious blood-vessel problems. With our patient the heart attacks she survived and the peripheral bleeding problems — bluish-red markings in the area of the toes, nose and fingers — all pointed towards the hawthorn mistletoe. In most cases the affected people are rather lean and excessively focused on their profession. They can scarcely talk about their feelings. They are only slightly given to fantasy and look upon life more from the aspect of their professional duties. The effectiveness of the hawthorn mistletoe is primarily recognizable by the thorough warming of the whole body, also on the surface — and by the increasing cordiality of the patients.

6. Metals Increase the Healing Force of Mistletoe

Alongside mistletoe, several metals are significant in the anthroposophical treatment of cancer, which has already been mentioned in many of the case studies in Chapter 5. At first glance this may not be readily understood. But the effects metals can have on people's bodies and state of mind has recently been brought to light by the discussion about mercury amalgam. It is obvious that with amalgam dental fillings tiny amounts of metallic substances are sluiced into the body, and over the course of time this can lead to serious cases of poisoning. In the amalgam, we are concerned with an alloy of mercury and many other metals, in particular copper, tin and silver. As a rule the amalgam does not cause poisoning directly — the resulting complaints are of the lingering and non-specific kind and are often considered doubtful from a scientific standpoint.

Some symptoms of amalgam poisoning are, however, uncontested: people become easily exhausted, increasingly irritable, lose memory function, are increasingly susceptible to allergens, suffer concentration problems, a diminished work capacity, sleep disorders, depression, headaches and become more susceptible to infections (especially in the mouth and throat) and chronic infections of the large intestine. These are also the preliminary symptoms of a cancerous disease. It thereby becomes clear that amalgam and cancer stand in a certain relationship to each other. In homeopathy a therapy with potentized metallic substances has long been an accepted method of treating chronic illnesses; anthroposophical medicine also treats cancer very successfully with differentiated use of metals.

Interestingly enough, metallic preparations are also used in one of the oldest systems of healing, namely in Tibetan medicine. Monk-doctors concoct their self-made plant medications and pills using mercury and/or silver preparations, according to ancient recipes. This tradition is continued in Dharamshala, the home of the exiled Dalai Lama.

The use of metals for healing sicknesses is therefore no esoteric invention of our time, but has deep roots worldwide. The sometimes positive, sometimes destructive force of metallic substances was therefore known to medicine long before Rudolf Steiner's mistletoe therapy. In his medical lecture cycle he expressly pointed out that when treating cancer the efficacy of mistletoe can be considerably increased with a supplementary metal therapy. He also specified the inner relationships that exist between the individual organs and certain metals: lead has a relationship with the spleen; tin with the liver; iron with the gall bladder; copper with the kidneys; gold with the heart; mercury with the lungs; silver with the urogenital organs; platinum with the pancreas.

So in order to achieve the maximum healing affect in mistletoe therapy it's not only important that the host tree on which the mistletoe grows corresponds to the particular human type, but also that the correct selection of metal be prescribed for the cancer patient. It's down to the skill of the doctor to recognize which metal can be of help to the patient. To do that he must be able to see, besides the similarities between the host tree and the personality of the patient, the connections between the patient's being and the particular characteristics of the metal. Not every metal is suitable for every type of human being.

Therefore before beginning a mistletoe therapy the doctor must find an analogy between the external appearance of the patient and his biography, and a certain metal. Only when this connection between the human and metallic qualities has been found can one combine the specific mistletoe treatment with a suitable metal therapy, and in this way achieve the optimum result for the cancer patient.

Lead — against the laming of life

Following the homeopathic principle of treating something with something similar, lead substances are suitable for patients whose life processes seem to be lamed. They are mostly emaciated people with deep wrinkles who appear devoid of strength and give the impression of being numbed and 'leaden.' This lameness also applies to their inner life of thoughts and feelings.

Patients speak extremely slowly and have a hard time formulating their thoughts. They frequently suffer from loss and impairment of memory. Their feelings are often poorly expressed. A characteristic often observed with leaden types of people, almost in contradiction to this heaviness, is a recurring desire to gamble, and a general tendency towards addiction (i.e. alcohol). Such people often feel a longing to do something forbidden. Becoming less able to stretch out the wrist and foot is a characteristic symptom of lead poisoning. Other striking symptoms are a withering away of the muscles, a rigidity in the blood vessels (the patient looks pale with high blood pressure) and a tendency towards chronic constipation. Frequently there's an insensitivity in certain skin areas, and patients suffer from infertility or impotence.

If one relates the symptoms described above to the carcinoma, then lead is, above all, an appropriate treatment for bone metastases, because it's in the bones that the life force of the patient seems to be most severely 'lamed.'

Iron — for the courage to fight for life

Iron is brought into a relationship with aggression, fighting and masculinity. The Latin name, *ferrum*, means to walk against, to approach, to turn towards someone, to undertake. In cancer therapy the prescription of iron substances makes sense when patients lack the fighting courage needed to take their destiny into their own hands. One also recognizes these patients from their tendency to be anaemic and become red with the slightest exertion. One must also consider iron when there has been a great loss of blood or with heavily bleeding tumours.

Patients who need iron mostly define themselves through their actions in life; they can only express their feelings with difficulty. Even when such people appear strong on the outside, they often have considerable weaknesses, particularly in speaking and walking. They are characterized by their pale skin and their great sensitivity, even to the slightest noise. Corresponding to the nature of iron, their headaches tend to be of the hammering kind. They can be ravenously hungry or completely lacking in appetite; often they cannot stand eating eggs. Iron types often complain of pain in their arms or shoulder joints.

When patients with cancer come down with feverish infections or pneumonia, the anthroposophical doctor will reinforce their mistletoe therapy with iron preparations. Like no other remedy, these give the patient a new courage for life and take away the fear of the tumour.

Gold — for finding one's own centre

Gold stands in relation to the human being as 'heaviness,' signifying melancholy and depression, which in desperation can sometimes even lead to suicide. With gold we have the polarity between inner and outer values. One often finds gold patients in leading positions in business, politics and other spheres of society. They almost always carry a lot of responsibility. They can be recognized by their compact build, with a bulbous nose, a choleric temperament, but properly dressed and well behaved. They are very much inclined towards the material things of life and need acknowledgment, a successful career and to be well off. On the other hand this striving for outer success often goes hand in hand with business worries; with failures and material problems they can sink into deepest depression, which can bring on a kind of death wish in them. Because of their one-sided direction in material life, they usually lack the courage to trust in a higher, perhaps divine guidance.

Gold patients frequently suffer from strokes, heart attacks, serious autoimmune diseases, skin diseases or cirrhosis of the liver. They complain of headaches that often occur around the head, as if below a crown. Gold patients' complaints always get worse at night. Bodily and spiritual movement works positively in these people — from dance, to meditation, to prayer, even loud weeping can do good as an inner movement.

It's apparent with gold patients that they are not calm within themselves, but that they have lost their centre. If 'laming' is a considerable aspect of lead, and 'lacking in strength' the effect of tin, then gold is characteristic for the absence of the 'inner sun.'

Copper — against cramping and guilt

Copper, the metal of Venus, is related to aesthetics and to feelings. In homeopathy it's primarily used to treat both cramping in both body and soul.

As a rule, copper patients have a strongly developed sense of duty. They achieve much, are disciplined and are acknowledged in society on account of their loving being. Nevertheless, they often suffer from guilty feelings and feel stifled. Because outwardly they always want to appear friendly and obliging, they become inwardly cramped. They often long for the secret fulfillment of wishes that are not in accord with social norms, or are even illegal. Because of their lack of courage copper people are often angry with themselves; their aggressive feelings can hardly find their way out, leaving the body in a state of cramp. The first indication of this condition is a grinding of the teeth. Already in infancy, soon after birth, stomach cramps can indicate a disturbed condition of copper in the body. Further symptoms are feverish or emotional cramps, convulsive twitching in various parts of the body, or bunions.

In the treatment of carcinomas, copper is always appropriate when a venous blockage has formed, or when, along with suffering from a tumour, one can see severe cramping in body and soul. Copper substances can also effectively support mistletoe therapy for breast cancer and carcinomas of the thyroid gland.

Mercury — for the right 'I–you' relationship

Mercury is perhaps one of the most difficult metals to understand. Historically it was used above all to treat syphilitic diseases; today it's mainly prescribed for diseases of the lymphatic system.

Patients with imbalanced internal mercury distribution are frequently recognized by their aggression. They are sure of their own judgments and don't like to be contradicted. Mercury patients live very intensely and feel the need to speak honestly about things that other people would prefer not to talk about: an attitude that can be hurtful and damaging to others. Therefore they can be difficult and uncomfortable to be around. This can even affect their relationship with their doctor, whom they often expect to agree unconditionally with their own evaluation of their illness, which can ultimately result in them discontinuing treatment.

Even the outer appearance of Mercury people can be deemed threatening — short hair, a shaved head, or being showily dressed. They sometimes suffer from extreme perspiration and give out an unpleasant body odour. They suffer in particular from sweating at night and from abscesses. They also typically have a tendency to salivate or have slimy stools (ulcerative colitis). Mercury influences the relationship between self and surroundings, which takes place in the body through the mucous membranes: in a figurative sense, through the 'I–you' relationship.

Phlegm-producing tumours or tumours that develop out of the mucous membranes mostly require treatment with mercury. This applies generally to all mucous membranes, but above all to the large intestine and the lungs.

Silver — against claustrophobia

According to Rudolf Steiner, silver or silver nitrate is the most important metal in the treatment of cancer. Silver and silver salts are proven remedies for pain and disturbances in the uterus, the ovaries and the testicles. Silver also has a connection with the larynx, and can be used for treating hoarseness, sore throats and laryngitis. Silver has been used to help ease swollen cartilage and hardening of the ligaments. One should also think of silver salts if the patient is frightened or anxious.

Silver types are characterized by compulsive behaviour. They are constantly afraid of making fools of themselves. Sometimes they are pursued by compulsive thoughts, for example, imagining that a building might suddenly collapse on top of them, or that they could get hit by a train. Fear of flying or of crowds are classic indications that the patient should be treated with silver preparations. The fears of these people arise from claustrophobic feelings: from being afraid of exams, to a fear of confined spaces or tunnels. Alongside these experiences of confinement, opposite feelings of expansion can occur, mostly perceived in the head, the stomach and in the ovaries.

However, the most frequently occurring experience of claustrophobia is reminiscent of the unconscious pre-birth experience of confinement followed by ejection through the birth canal; consequently it's not surprising that carcinomas related to the vagina almost always have a connection to silver. Cancers that occur in silver people have often been caused by birth trauma, an artificially induced birth, or feelings of claustrophobia that arose later in life.

But besides silver, two other 'silvery' metals are also important: platinum, a kind of 'iron-silver' (for carcinomas of the pancreas), and uranium, the 'silver of old age,' which is used against abdominal ulcers in the form of an internal radiation therapy. However the corresponding preparations are forbidden in Germany and may only be obtained in some countries.

Tin — against exhaustion and apathy

While lead in the human being has a laming effect, tiredness and a deep chronic weakness are characteristic of tin. Along with this, tin shows a strong relationship to the chest and to weaknesses of the respiratory system, also to tuberculosis and its aftermath. Characteristics are difficulty in breathing, especially while walking, or a rather loose cough with a sweetish expectorant. The patient feels weak in the chest when speaking.

Too much tin makes people's hands and wrists feel weak when writing. The larynx is often involved: singers, for example, then complain about pains in the neck and elsewhere when they cough. Typical tin symptoms in the head region are pressure pains in the forehead; if they occur in the back of the head they are more likely caused by lead.

It's typical of a lack of tin that ailments start around 10 am, get stronger until about 4 pm, then gradually subside again. Patients who need tin have a great longing to lie down and be restful. They don't feel very comfortable in the company of other people. People with too little tin tend to start work on tasks without completing them; they often feel tired and sleepy. They often lapse into sadness (notably women suffering from premenstrual tension) and into a powerless state of apathy and being fed up with life, often linked to anxiety. In unusual cases the lack of tin leads to a sullen state of mind or to conscious malice.

Tin is thought to influence the development of physical strength and the formation of the organs. Consequently the contribution of tin is indicated when an organ has become weak and powerless. This applies especially to liver carcinomas, but also to cancer of the larynx and of the respiratory system.

7. Mistletoe Inoculation Against Cancer

As a doctor in a clinic I have to deal with cancer patients every day, with their pain and grief, with their hopes and disappointments. Whoever works with these people, from those who are recovering to those who die, has to be especially careful and consciously responsible with their prognoses and promises of healing, in order not to awaken false expectations. But my positive experiences with optimized mistletoe therapies lead towards new avenues in cancer treatment, and they even guide me to this make this thesis: people with a predisposition for cancer can be 'inoculated' with a preventative treatment according to the principles of optimized mistletoe therapy, in order to prevent the later outbreak of the disease.

Of course with this prophylaxis it is not a matter of inoculation in the customary sense, in which people are given an inoculation that is produced by the thousand. It will rather be an entirely individual mixture of substances that the doctor puts together on the basis of his experience with optimized mistletoe therapy, and with which he injects the person threatened by cancer. The principles of this preventative treatment are the same as the mistletoe therapy for a person who is already sick. Although the inoculation for each particular case is individually prepared, such an inoculation for cancer requires a great deal from the doctor. It is just not enough to simply recognize the symptoms and to follow through with an inoculation, or to give a well-tested inoculation to a small child.

In cancer prevention the doctor must grasp the individual in their entirety and in addition must know the characteristic features of mistletoe trees and of metals as they have been described in this book. Only then is it possible to mix an effective inoculation. This requires much time and knowledge, but the substances that make up the inoculation, which is specific to the individual patient, are relatively cheap; there is certainly no comparison with the enormous costs required for the standard treatment of cancer diseases today.

My thesis that one can inoculate people early on against cancer is based on three considerations:

1. The scientifically proven fact that mistletoes strengthen the human immune system and destroy tumour cells which are present.
2. The opinion shared by doctors of all persuasions that a cancerous disease does not arise from one week to the next, but almost always has a prior history.
3. A mistletoe inoculation, even if unsuccessful, does not produce any negative side effects.

Doctors and researchers know today that cancer gradually develops in the body and soul of a human being up to twenty years before it actually breaks out. If one compares the long time period in which the disease develops to the statistic that three quarters of all first illnesses occur after the age of sixty, then the question arises: what is special about the phase of life in which cancer insinuates itself, between the mid-forties and sixty? Why does middle age present such a great danger? Why does a carcinoma develop in some people and not in others, in smokers for example, although their life circumstances are comparable? And what can one do to prevent the outbreak of cancer?

When after his mid-forties an apparently healthy person shows symptoms that may lead to developing a cancerous disease, I am firmly convinced he can be helped with a prophylactic 'mistletoe inoculation.' Of course, it's not yet possible for me to scientifically prove this prognosis; for that my knowledge is too recent. But my experience so far with patients who have a pre-cancerous condition (an alteration in the tissues which is recognizable as a preliminary stage of cancer) confirms this thesis. In the meantime I have treated numerous middle-aged people who showed a tendency towards developing cancer with optimized mistletoe therapy, and the signs which indicated cancer almost always promptly disappeared.

What happens in the pre-cancerous state?

In conventional medicine it is still disputed whether a preliminary condition from which cancer develops, with recognizable criteria, actually exists. This excludes, of course, the classical risk factors, such as smoking, bad diet, too little exercise and a family history of developing cancer.

The connection between psychological trauma and cancer is now taken more seriously, since leading oncologists have proven that there is a close correlation between cancers and past experiences of social separation — for example, the death of a spouse, a divorce, or serious illnesses or depression.

With this knowledge, occurrences during the pre-cancerous period take on a deep significance, because such cancer-causing factors can be removed or minimized using preventative inoculation measures based on mistletoe therapy.

However, before we go into the details of a cancer inoculation, let's focus on the pre-cancerous period: in our case on the aforementioned phase of life between the mid-forties and sixty, during which, according to statistics, three out of four subsequent cancer illnesses arise. In Germany alone 300,000 people are afflicted by this every year.

The life of an individual is something unique; no one else leads an identical life. Nevertheless in all cultures and at all times, experience shows that the life rhythms of all humans between birth and death have much in common. This recognition even led to a life model based on observations made from time immemorial: the 'rhythm of seven.' It says that, starting at birth, the human being enters into a new phase of life every seven years, a development which brings him new experiences and attitudes every time. Modern psychoanalysis — from C. G. Jung to the psycho-oncologists of the present time — has extensively confirmed the developments described in this ancient rhythm of seven.

Essentially it's a matter of observing how the human being's life rhythm stands in relation to the rhythms of creation surrounding him, which influence his life: the alternation of day and night which results from the rotation of the earth and the course of the sun; the effects of the planets, which are reflected for instance in the forces of the moon and its influence on people, animals and plants; the course of the seasons of the year. The human being's life rhythm is obviously bound together with a cosmic order. For our considerations, however, the question that interests us concerning the seven-year cycle is: what happens to the human being during the pre-cancerous stage in the phase of life between mid-forties and sixty?

It can be established that this is a typical time for gaining new insights and spiritual perspectives. People feel that their striving efforts are gradually coming to rest, that life no longer consists of conflicts, of victory or defeat. In the first half of life the emphasis lay principally on externals: professional career, owning a house, cars and vacations, parties and events — together with raising a family, children growing up and a circle of friends.

During middle-age, on the other hand, there is almost always a major shift: people are confronted with life-changing events. Often parents and old friends die during this time, quite often a marriage breaks up, children leave home and go their own ways, careers become more demanding, with a change of job or threat of redundancy — and people notice the first signs of wear and tear on body and soul. It's a time when the first serious experiences of loss make people aware of their own limitations. From the mid-forties on, people can feel that life has withheld a great many things and they start to wonder why.

But with the background of such experiences they are also able to connect with their inner selves more easily, to become more thoughtful, to open themselves up to spirituality, perhaps to faith — in any case, to tread their path more slowly. They become aware that growth is not endless, but is equally based on becoming and passing away.

The strong tensions which up to now determined life and success gradually diminish, the combative element yields to a calmer attitude — and people become aware of relationships to which, until now, they had scarcely paid attention. Now they can look upon life with greater peace and from a greater distance, without allowing themselves to become so easily upset. Personal aims at the threshold of the second half of life are directed more towards the inner self, and the gaze is directed away from the earth and to something higher.

People are more ready to help others, and now from honest conviction and no longer from calculation, as may have previously been the case. And so it is perfectly natural that they no longer occupy themselves with their own destiny and the purpose of life. Fundamentally these are the first steps on the way to wisdom.

Many people, however, don't see this entirely natural midlife change as an opportunity, and react in the wrong way. They refuse to look within themselves, and begin to flee. They often throw themselves even more violently into the outer world and forcefully try to improve everything. Along with this they become inconsiderate, dogmatic and often even tyrannical. Business people cling on to their positions and refuse to accept generational changes. They believe they are irreplaceable and must continue to fight on. Some escape into restlessness, throw away their previous lifestyle and fanatically flit from one experiment to the next. Still others cling like iron to their existing attitudes and refuse to accept change or renewal, becoming rigid and numb.

Often such disturbances between the mid-forties and sixty are not perceived at all, because people at this age are still physically fit and healthy. Their good physical condition masks the fact that at this stage of life they should be gradually turning away from material things towards soul and spiritual development. If they learn to overcome their emotions, if they disregard their spiritual development, if they continue to be incited and driven, if they do not transform the old pressure to succeed into greater calmness of mind, and if stress continues to embitter their life and they cannot find inner peace, people lose their rhythm, their balance and their centre. Whoever disregards this midlife change upsets the natural rhythm of life and opens the gates for the invasion of all kinds of diseases; cancer now finds its fertile soil.

In psycho-oncology these mis-developments have been noted, though of course only in retrospect. They show the inclination for cancer long before there is any evidence of tissue changes. But unfortunately clinging to conventional certainties is stronger in many people than the readiness for change, for the step into the next stage of life. In such cases feelings and fears are not freely expressed and consciously worked through, but are forced down into the subconscious. The thread of an individually structured life can then easily break; loss of purpose, lack of perspective and aversion close off the way forward. The inner forces that are lying fallow can break out into abnormal organic growth, and the will to live becomes a will to destroy. Life energy that is not transformed into meaningful thinking, feeling and action can degenerate and grow into carcinomas.

When to inoculate?

During middle-age everyone should stand back and reflect on their life, without rose- tinted glasses, but openly and self-critically. The disturbances of body and soul which they may then discover can help to rearrange their life — above all in the emotional area, in order to strengthen their self-healing forces. This increase in energy will also enable the immune system to remove cancer cells that are trying to secure a place somewhere in the body.

Of course, it's not always easy to analyze the state of one's own feelings and draw the right conclusions from them. But from the mid-forties onwards, stress and a disturbed life rhythm show up in many bodily reactions, which ought to be a signal that something is not right. We have already mentioned these reactions throughout the book and will summarize them again here.

The following midlife symptoms can be precursors of a later cancer disease:

Constant freezing or shivering because the body is not warm enough. Normal body temperature is 37°C (98.4°F). If it is constantly below that and one often has cold hands and feet, then something is wrong. In the evening body temperature should be slightly higher than in the morning, by at least 0.5°C (1°F)

Tiredness, often to the point of exhaustion, is an indication that life rhythm has been badly disturbed. This symptom is often expressed through a lack of enthusiasm for work, for social engagements and for sex.

Insomnia, difficulty in falling asleep and frequent awakening during the night prevent the human being from recovering through a healthy sleep and gathering strength for the following day; the lost rhythm of sleeping and waking works negatively on body and soul.

Constant night sweats are a sign that the state of body and/or soul has become disturbed.

The increase of warts shows that something is not in order.

Attacks of dizziness, especially when getting up in the morning or when moving quickly, should also not be ignored.

Premature ageing is another warning signal, showing that the biological and actual ages are no longer in balance. This is true of smokers, whose yellowish skin is often a sign of premature aging.

People who smoke more than ten cigarettes a day are especially in danger. The connection between smoking and cancer is no longer disputed by anyone.

Psychological traumas, which happen to many people during middle-age, can significantly increase their susceptibility to cancer. Among these are the death of a spouse, relation or good friend, divorce, serious illness, financial problems, career changes, being made redundant, and any events that put a similar burden on the mind.

Restlessness, and haste in not allowing one's own thoughts, feelings and actions — as well as those of others — to run their course, but constantly interfering: these are indications of a disrupted life rhythm.

People do no good to their immune system when they are overweight, get hardly any exercise and eat poorly: too little fruit, vegetables or fibre, too much fat and fast food. A tendency for overweight people to be more susceptible to colon and breast cancer was observed.

No one should get overwrought if they notice one or other of these symptoms in themselves. It would be absurd to constantly watch yourself like a hypochondriac and allow the slightest hint of a problem to stop you enjoying life. Any single one of these symptoms is a long way from being a harbinger of cancer. Only a noticeable accumulation of them can point to a threatening condition and a danger of cancer. Therefore any middle-aged person who notices several such symptoms should pay attention to them. If the person is also experiencing disruptions in their life rhythm, as described in relation to the seven-year cycle — and if beyond that there is genetic history of cancer in the family — then such observations should be taken seriously. As a precaution, in such cases, it's advisable to consult a doctor who has training in natural healing. In the appendix (p. 161) we have listed the addresses of several institutions who can give information about finding such doctors.

It must then be decided, in consultation with the doctor, if a preventative cancer inoculation is necessary. If the answer is yes, then such a course of treatment will begin. It is carried out following the same principles as an optimized mistletoe therapy used for treating existing carcinomas. The doctor must first search for the analogies between the person and the mistletoe host tree. The potentized substances of the chosen mistletoe will usually then be enriched with metal substances, which are also appropriate to the patient's being. And sometimes this is supplemented with homeopathic remedies.

Therefore the cancer inoculation consists of a combination of mistletoe extracts, metal substances and anthroposophical-homeopathic remedies, and it's an individual mixture for this particular patient. The patient's biography and the relationship of their being to certain mistletoes and metals alone determine the composition of the inoculation.

I found in my clinical work with preventative inoculations that particular mistletoes are especially helpful for treating certain kinds of damage to the body. It turns out that mistletoe inoculations not only have an anti-cancerous effect, but that they can heal a whole series of diseases that are not typically considered to influence the development of cancer.

Lime mistletoe, for example, has positive effects not only on passive and active smokers, but also on people who have family conflicts.

People in danger of getting cancer, who present a perfect outward façade, but are inwardly hardened and petrified from being abused in body or soul as children, can be helped by almond mistletoe. They can often be recognized by a tendency for basalioma (a harmless skin disease) or for numerous liver spots early in life.

Ash mistletoe is used above all when a state of exhaustion appears in rather thin, athletic patients who are in a pre-cancerous state.

Oak mistletoe is suitable for vigorous personalities whose immune system has been weakened by heavy blows of destiny.

Apple-tree mistletoe is the most important for prophylaxis of the digestive system, especially with overweight patients who have a tendency to eat voraciously. Often these people have previously had diabetes or metabolic syndrome, in which various complaints succeed one another.

A birch mistletoe inoculation is suitable for thin people who report a lack of sexual desire or weakness in their kidney-bladder system.

For autoimmune diseases, in which faulty cells within the body attack their own cells, pine mistletoe is the best inoculation, especially for slender people who have thyroid problems, have noticed an increased development of warts, or complain of rheumatic ailments.

Maple mistletoe is suitable for people suffering from strong fluctuations in their blood sugar level, and especially for those with a repeated tendency for hypoglycaemia (very low blood sugar level).

Willow mistletoe is now practically recognized as a remedy for fibromyalgia when the muscles and ligaments of the arms and shoulders have become hardened, or for pain in the bones and joints, including rheumatic diseases. In such cases therapy with willow mistletoe should be begun early on to prevent carcinomas.

Fir mistletoe is preferred for older people, especially for patients who are constantly cold, which is typical for a pre-cancerous condition.

Elm mistletoe is particularly suitable for heavy smokers, or those who are also exposed to other poisons in the environment or partake of them to excess.

Poplar mistletoe is an effective remedy for all early recognizable carcinomas of the prostate. One should begin with poplar mistletoe injections when the tumour marker level is slightly elevated, but not yet at the point of requiring an operation.

The inoculation

As soon as the doctor has determined the symptoms and knows the analogies between the patient, the host tree of the mistletoe and a characteristic metal, the actual inoculation can begin. The inoculation is injected beneath the skin of the abdomen once a week. As mentioned in Chapter 2, the patient can also administer this simple injection himself, as is done by diabetics who inject insulin themselves. After the seventh injection there is a break of one week, which is followed by a second series of seven weekly injections under the skin of the abdomen as before.

After only a few injections a reddening often occurs around the injection spot and/or there is a significant rise in body temperature, the desired 'mistletoe fever,' which disappears again after three days at the most. These are signs that the injected material is already working. This high fever, which can reach 40°C (104°F), is of course the aim of the cancer prophylaxis, because it warms up the individual cells just as it does the whole body.

It is also possible for these symptoms not to appear, even though the effects are taking place in the body. Patients usually feel that the inoculation is taking hold in body and soul after a few days: they have strength all day long, sleep well again, feel inwardly warmed up and experience a greater joy of life. The active substances now strengthen the immune system, develop the self-healing forces, and at the same time destroy any eventual cancer cells that could have formed somewhere in the body.

As a rule the inoculation treatment of fourteen injections is completed after four months, and the inoculation costs around €100.

Case studies

Here are some examples of mistletoe inoculations from my clinical work:

Prostate at risk

The patient was a 62-year-old business executive whose profession made great demands on him and who carried a lot of responsibility. He was big and strong with a fighting spirit, great will power and fully preserved sexuality. He ate well and worked out regularly in a gym. He felt physically very fit, his weight remained constant and he had no night sweats; only his blood pressure had been too high for some years.

Then at a check-up the tumour marker showed significantly increased PSA values and prostate cancer was suspected.

However, the man was afraid that an eventual operation would cause him to become incontinent and weaken his sexuality, so he refused any further conventional treatment and wanted to try mistletoe therapy.

Because the man had the physique of an athlete with a great fighting strength, as well as the masculine location of the potential cancer (the prostate), and because of the high arterial blood pressure, I prescribed an inoculation treatment with oak mistletoe.

The patient returned after three months. In the meantime he had received a series of oak mistletoe injections, without having experienced any noticeable change in temperature. However, since receiving the mistletoe injections his blood pressure had become normal, meaning that the medication prescribed for hypertension could soon be completely stopped. Along with this, the tumour marker levels had reduced by half, and the possibility of an operation is no longer being discussed.

Oak mistletoe is definitely related to people with pronounced masculine characteristics: that is with excessive emphasis on their work life and sport activities. Therefore the oak mistletoe is almost exclusively appropriate for men.

Uterine fibroid (myoma)

A 45-year-old woman was diagnosed with swellings in her uterus some years ago. The patient had withdrawn herself from her husband, her social circle and work. She avoided other people. Outwardly she appeared shapeless, stout and phlegmatic. In recent years her weight had increased from 70kg (155 lb) to almost 100 kg (220 lb). This was evidently due to her passion for food, primarily because of her ravenous appetite for sweets and candies — she could hardly control herself in this. She was highly dissatisfied with her life. She conducted her business, a confectioner's shop, listlessly and the relationship with her husband was only one of convenience. Even her own children could not console her for the lack of meaning in her life.

The myoma, a harmless tumour, in addition to the patient's ongoing obsession with food, her ravenous appetite, her constant bingeing on sweets, but also her listlessness and misjudgments of other people, together with her corpulent figure, were for me typical signs indicating the apple tree and its mistletoe. The patient therefore received an apple-tree mistletoe inoculation.

At the examination three months later the woman already felt much better. Her facial expressions as well as her body movements were more mobile, although she had not yet lost any weight. She said that she was now more motivated to organize her own life and took an interest again in the world around her; she had become more aware of her rejection of her husband. Her ravenous appetite for sweets was almost completely gone. The myoma in her uterus however was still unchanged.

Three months later the woman came to the practice completely changed. She now weighed 10 kg (22 lb) less, and she had taken herself and her destiny into her own hands. Compared with before, she appeared happier and more structured in her facial expressions. She said that one day she had suddenly felt as if 'a lump' in her gut had dissolved.

In her case the potentized mistletoe seemed to have led to her becoming conscious of her own self. It can only be surmised, therefore, whether a threatening cancerous illness was prevented. The apple-tree mistletoe is the most important mistletoe for the colon, since most of the carcinomas of the large intestine are caused by poor nourishment.

Cancer in the family, autoimmune deficiency, exhaustion

The 48-year-old lean, wiry patient has never properly regained her strength after suffering from glandular fever (Pfeiffer's disease) three years ago. Until then she was fully occupied in her profession and took care of the whole household, including three children. After work she even took part in sports.

But then she also came down with an autoimmune deficiency of the thyroid gland. After only a few hours of physical work the woman was now completely exhausted and had to rest. The numerous examinations by various doctors and in hospitals could not determine the cause of her affliction. A two-year homeopathic therapy had also not achieved the desired healing, although in between there was always some slight improvement.

In our clinic the woman complained of feeling constantly cold and shivering — and we learned that her mother had died of a breast carcinoma.

One sensed a strong (angry) force in the woman, which she had internalized. Her characteristics and symptoms indicated the ash: a lean figure, but at the same time filled with strength, with high demands in her profession and household, with a family history of cancer, with an autoimmune deficiency and instances of great exhaustion — all characteristic signs of a pre-cancerous condition. I therefore prescribed an ash mistletoe inoculation for the patient.

After a treatment of two months she experienced a definite improvement in body temperature; she no longer felt freezing and had strength for the whole day. Since then she has been stable and her thyroid gland has functioned normally.

What the oak mistletoe is for the man, the ash mistletoe appears to be for the woman: a medication for feminine, athletic women who frequently overload themselves with the self-imposed duties of family and profession.

Fibromyalgia

A fifty-year-old patient had been complaining for years about increasing pain in the region of the shoulder and neck, which also spread down into her arms. Three years earlier, an orthopedist has diagnosed a case of fibromyalgia — painful hardening of the connective tissue between tendons and muscles — not cancer.

The lean woman suffered from shooting pains whenever she raised her arm above the horizontal. She acted as if numbed, also in her facial expression, movements and speech. She ascribed the probable cause of these symptoms to life developments which had become a great psychological burden: the business that she had built up with her husband was no longer profitable, so she saw herself forced to look for other work.

The apparent blockage of movement in the joints, but also the numbness and the psychological as well as the physical inflexibility of the woman were typical symptoms indicating the willow. On the basis of this finding I carried out a willow mistletoe inoculation for this patient.

After just a few weeks she was better. Her pain and mood improved visibly, the woman felt relaxed and full of the joy of living. Before, she had tended to look at the world in a negative way, but now she could enjoy the good things of life. She had left her husband's business and found another field of work. In spite of the burdens due to this change, her ailments had not returned: on the contrary, she could hardly feel pain any more.

A year later, the woman, who was now free of complaints, confessed her sorrow to the doctor. She had been considering separation from her husband for twenty years, but could not make herself take this step. She felt that her husband was too inaccurate and inexact in his work, and did not take her fears for their security seriously. She was now happy that she didn't have to work with him any more and had found another job. She decided to finally separate from her husband as soon as their daughter has completed her studies.

The willow mistletoe is a good remedy for fibromyalgia, as well as for rheumatic ailments and helps against chronic problems at the muscle-tendon connections, above all in the shoulders and the cervical (neck) region of the spinal column; it also helps to treat cancer of the kidneys and leukaemia: that is to say, whenever it is a matter of tissue regeneration.

Depression and impotence

In the following case, the patient's illness did not yet show any actual indication of cancer, but possibly a dangerous prior condition.

A fifty-year-old manager diagnosed with 'depression and impotence' had been working for a large firm until two years ago. He had been traveling a lot, and since these numerous business trips continually kept him apart from his family he had decided to work independently, which didn't turn out well. During the first year, the man became increasingly depressed. He no longer felt well, he saw his ability to perform disappearing, and he had trouble with his sexual performance and no longer felt able to deal with the marital relationship. He now seldom had sex with his wife; he just had sporadic erotic fantasies in his dreams. The patient appeared to have slowed down mentally and physically and his speech was impaired. Many of the patient's characteristics and symptoms indicated the birch mistletoe.

The birch stands for purity, also chastity, so there is an analogy to lean, spiritual people with a religious background. But in its character it also corresponds to those people who involuntarily live according to the law of chastity — the birch mistletoe can help them. Apart from that, the patient showed the symptoms that indicate birch mistletoe therapy: tiredness, lack of desire, loneliness.

The patient's career break at around the age of fifty, as well as his feelings of emptiness, also indicated a connection with the birch and to the metal tin. Therefore I prescribed a birch mistletoe therapy and in addition the patient was given tin in homeopathic doses.

After three months the businessman was transformed. He was much livelier, his impotence problems had completely gone, he felt altogether well and had strength and joy in his life once again.

This case provides an example of how the birch mistletoe, as well as tin, can be of central importance in helping patient's who suffer life crises in their forties and fifties. Tin helped with the psychological consequences of the career break and the emptiness of the soul; birch mistletoe helped to remedy the impotence. However birch mistletoe injections can produce (pseudo)allergic reactions, therefore the physician must be very careful and start with low potency levels.

8. Transferring the Mistletoe's Wisdom

The history of mankind is rich in examples of wisdom transferred from the natural world. Cosmic events, happenings in nature, the observation of animals and plants — from these, human beings have always found stimulation for their own lives. The bird was a model for the building of aeroplanes; the hull of a modern tanker is like the body of a dolphin; gardeners take account of the moon to improve the growth of plants: examples of how human beings have learned from creation could be pursued in manifold ways.

Nowadays, however, there are increasing signs that nature is making a stand against the human being's delusion of omnipotence; the eruption of volcanoes, hurricanes, tidal waves and earthquakes remind us of some of the boundaries we have arrogantly crossed.

Another sign from nature is a development that has been occurring for some years, almost unnoticed, alongside the destruction of forests: the almost explosive growth of mistletoe. In many cities there is hardly a tree that is not covered with mistletoe — they nest in the boughs and branches like spherical abscesses.

Anyone who does not believe that nature and creation are accidental products which have arisen by themselves without any recognizable purpose — but that they are a gigantic network of interdependent relationships — would ask himself the question: why does mistletoe connect itself with dying trees right now? Mistletoe actually seems to be sending us a message that can help us at this critical time: warmth heals human beings!

In the battle against cancer, mistletoe mysteriously kindles a 'fire' (mistletoe fever) in the cells, which inflames the self-healing forces of the human being. Like a warm cloak, the active substances of this magic plant wrap themselves around the cell and awaken it to new life. The return to joy and courage in life, initiated by mistletoe, strengthens cancer patients: this wonderful wisdom transfer from plant to human being gives patients new strength and stimulates them to conduct their lives in a self-determined way.

Such thoughts are no mere utopian whims, but have long since proven themselves as successful realities in modern cancer treatment. A study by Dr Grossarth-Maticek of 10,000 patients (see also p. 154) proved beyond doubt that 'self-regulation,' namely the freeing of life from too many outside influences, is perhaps the most powerful healing factor in human beings. Mistletoe can make a decisive contribution to this — and furthermore, mistletoe often gives the impulse to change, to turn one's life around. Then the active substances of the mistletoe are transformed into a spiritual process: they restore the patients' unity of body and soul and strengthen their life forces.

Mistletoe can also play an important role for our gradually ageing population. Like no other plant, it can provide youthful forces, which help older people by giving them courage throughout the second half of life. One can see the effect of mistletoe working when, from within themselves, people feel the impulse to think about their life's plan and perhaps carry it out differently. Along with this, it may result in a more cheerful disposition and even activate a flagging sex life. In every way the mistletoe brings back the joy of living!

In a metaphorical sense it can become an aphrodisiac which kindles a love for the surrounding world, so that wonderful relationships awaken and grow with other human beings, and with nature. In a preventative way, it can develop into a kind of 'divine childhood,' causing 'spiritual children' to grow in the form of new ideas about life — instead of tumours and their metastases.

But the healing message of mistletoe not only concerns the individual human being, but our whole society. In the wealthy western countries a value system, tried and tested over many centuries, is currently disintegrating: virtues such as friendship, love of one's neighbour, solidarity, fidelity and understanding for the weakness of others are being increasingly crowded out by egotism and the irresponsible struggle to earn money. All other matters are subordinate to commercial aims, such as rationalization and globalization. This one-sided aim for maximum profits will lead to unbridled economic growth, which in the long run will destroy the state organism because it undermines the value system and drives the country to ruin due to ever rising unemployment. What happens in society is similar to the occurrence of cancer in the body: the unbridled growth is the mark of a carcinoma-like process. The cancer epidemic rages not only in the human being, but has long since also infected society.

It is significant that young people express their greatest admiration with the word 'cool.' But the cooling off of feeling and the often icy relationships that have arisen among people are not good for us. We have been sacrificed to a means of progress, which in many ways has not proved to be a blessing.

Perhaps mistletoe is also trying to pass on this message: just as mistletoe heals by warming the damaged cells and therefore the human being, similarly modern societies seem to need warmth for their healing.

Per arborem mortui,
per arborem vivificati

By the tree brought to death
By the tree given life again.

This is a quotation from Venantius Fortunatus, a follower of St Augustine. It refers to the Christian story of creation. Adam and Eve disobeyed God's command and ate from the tree of knowledge. Therefore they were driven out of paradise and had to die — and all mankind after them. Only through Jesus Christ, who died on a wooden cross, was the ability to overcome death given back to them.

This symbolism of transformation, which we meet in other religions and in many wisdom teachings, is also found in the mistletoe: its indwelling strength, which is further strengthened by the living sap of the host tree, is carried over to sick human beings and helps them to raise up the tree of life within themselves again.

Appendix

What causes cancer?

The formation of cancer involves 'oncogenes,' which cause morbid changes to take place in the cells. In the body of the human being 100 billion cells have joined together to form the tissues and organs, and they are constantly renewing themselves by splitting in two innumerable times. In order that these cell divisions proceed faultlessly, nature has implanted a complex regulatory system in the human body that balances the dying off of cells and their renewal in the right way.

However, when the human being's immune system is no longer functioning properly, 'carcinogens,' i.e. cancer-promoting agents (those in tobacco smoke and food, ultra-violet and ionizing radiation, certain viruses) can disturb the cells' equilibrium. And that can lead to individual cells becoming completely unbalanced and multiplying, at the expense of healthy cells, and growing into malignant tumours. Often these degenerate cells travel to other parts of the body in the bloodstream or the lymph nodes, and there they create — often far from their origin — 'daughter tumours,' known as 'metastases.'

Cancer appears in many varieties — around one hundred different carcinomas are known in medicine; some kinds of cancer grow very slowly and do not produce metastases, others positively explode: in leukaemia and lymphoma the disease appears without any tumours.

Insights and statistics

People can get cancer at any time of life. However, the danger increases with age, for example carcinoma of the prostate is a typical disease of older men. Survival rates vary a great deal with the different diseases. Children with leukaemia, young men with prostate cancer, people with lip and skin cancer have a very good chance of getting better. Even for malignant tumours of the colon and breast, survival rates have risen considerably in recent years. On the other hand, the prognosis for people diagnosed with cancer of the pancreas or the lungs is less hopeful, although even in these serious cases, improvement and sometimes even a cure, is possible.

But the unnecessarily high mortality rate of cancer sufferers is not only due to a lack of medical knowledge, but to the patients themselves, many of whom ignore risk factors and take too little responsibility for their own health. We have known for a long time, and been told in books, newspapers, radio and on television, that smoking alone is responsible for almost thirty per cent of all cancer illnesses which result in death; smoking not only affects the mouth cavity, the aesophagus, the larynx and the lungs, but also the pancreas, the bladder and in women the cervix. Most people know this and smoke in spite of it. Even the enormous price increases of cigarettes and the warning on the packets 'smoking kills' does not discourage smokers from their habit. In Europe 650,000 people die each year from the consequences of their nicotine addiction — almost always with great sorrow for those concerned, and putting enormous burdens on our healthcare systems.

It's the same with eating habits. Studies unmistakably show that in almost half of cancer cases, poor diet and being overweight are contributing factors. People who, despite knowing this, continue to eat and drink without following a few sensible ground rules — more fibre, less saturated fat, more vitamins, more fresh fruit and vegetables — must know that they are running a great risk of cancer, and should not be surprised if one day their body no longer has the strength to prevent the outbreak of this disease.

Working conditions can also be partly responsible for some cancer illnesses: it is estimated that they contribute to one in ten cases. One need only think of miners constantly breathing in dust, or unhygienic working places that expose employees to dangers or environmental poisons. Also managers whose life rhythm has become unbalanced because of stress must face the fact that their immune system is weakened all the time, and will eventually lose the fight against substances which bring on cancer.

In Germany pathogens and viruses (in the case of liver cancer) are responsible for about five per cent of cancer cases. In cases of stomach cancer, infection by the bacterium *Helicobacter pylori* is very likely and, in recent cases, has frequently been found.

The increasingly detailed knowledge about human genetics shows that one out of every ten cancer illnesses is attributable to a genetic predisposition. No wonder then that an unusually large number of cancer illnesses appear in some family histories. With malignant carcinomas of the eye, the intestines, the breast and the ovaries, one can almost always assume that there is an inherited predisposition.

Cancer illnesses vary according to sex: statistics show that there are significant differences in new illnesses between men and women each year. Prostate cancer is most common in men (20 %), followed by cancer in the intestines and the lungs (16 % each). In women breast cancer is the most common (25 %), followed by cancers of the intestines (18 %). All other carcinomas are far behind at 5 % or less.

The death statistics show a different order. There lung cancer is the biggest killer at almost 30 %, followed by intestinal cancers at 13 % and prostate cancer at 10 %. However, in women, the new cases of illness are identical with the actual number of deaths. Breast cancer leads the way not only with new cases but with causes of death at 18 %, followed by cancer of the intestines at 15 % and lung cancer at 10 %.

It is important, however, to be clear that statistics about cures, survival rates and deaths reflect the past. This is also true for new cases and mortality rates. The figures that are currently available can only reflect the past, and are not necessarily accurate — due to advances in medicine — for the present or for future developments.

Anyone diagnosed with cancer will, of course, want to find out about the most relevant therapies for treating their illness. This is first of all best achieved by consultations with doctors. To supplement this, we will briefly introduce the most frequently used therapeutic methods, arranged in alphabetical order. We have put them in two groups: conventional and complimentary treatments.

Conventional cancer treatments

Chemotherapy

In chemotherapy the patient is treated with cytostatics, which are supposed to check the excessive growth of the degenerate cancer cells. Cytostatics are poisons which destroy a cell at the moment of division. But unfortunately they not only destroy cancer cells, but also parts of healthy tissue.

The discovery of chemotherapy as a weapon against cancer is actually derived from military experience. Chemotherapy was developed after the Second World War, based on the knowledge of the devastating effect mustard gas has on people, which gave the idea to use cell poisons against carcinomas. Since then cell poisons have led to a murderous war in the body and soul of the human being.

Astounding results have been achieved with some cancers (leukaemia and lymphoma), so this radical therapy is justified despite the very considerable side effects. However with chemotherapy we come to a parting of ways. In the most recent studies, at any rate, there are increasing doubts about the healing effect of these poison cures. We know that cell poisons, often prescribed as the last resort, worsen the patient's quality of life dramatically. But what has recently been found is that, apparently, they hardly ever bring about a lengthening of the patient's life. Critics even claim the advancements in chemotherapy lie only in lessening the side effects which it has itself caused, in other words chemotherapy advances have not led to any improvement of life-expectancy.

This assessment does not appear to be merely an outsider's opinion. An increasing number of doctors would decline chemotherapy treatment themselves. Thus the maintenance of a large and expensive stock of cytostatics by the pharmaceutical industry becomes an increasingly greater risk. Some rethinking appears to be urgently required, not only for scientific and financial reasons, but above all in the interest of the patients.

Hormone therapy

Today it is known that the growth of certain carcinomas is dependent on hormones. Depending on the location of the disease, anti-hormonal preparations can so alter the hormone distribution in the body that the malignant tumour recedes or that the development of metastases is prevented. The current state of hormone therapy for cancer has been thoroughly described by the cancer research centre in Heidelberg; this information is the basis of the description which follows.

Hormones, as the body's signalling substances, have a decisive influence on the food assimilation process of the human being. The hormones produced in various glands arrive, through the blood, at their place of activity, where they 'dock' and give rise to a chain of reactions. The growth of some cancer cells is also guided by hormones — and conversely a hormone blockade can prevent the growth of tumour cells or at least reduce it. Such an anti-hormone therapy has proven itself above all with cancer of the breast and uterus as well as for prostate cancer. With the former, the female hormone oestrogen promotes growth; with prostate cancer, it comes from the male hormone testosterone. This growth-promoting effect can be avoided in a number of ways. Likewise the production of those particular hormones can be prevented by surgically removing the location where they originate, or by making them 'passive' with medication. Alternatively it is possible to block the action of the hormones in the affected cells with special antigens. These substances hem in the cancer cells without however interfering with the original purposeful task of the growth hormones.

In breast cancer prior to the end of menopause, the still active ovaries are eliminated as the source of oestrogen. Formerly this was done by surgical removal or by radiation; today it is possible to suppress the oestrogen formation with medication. During this therapy the ovaries stop producing oestrogen, so the woman experiences an artificial menopause. By discontinuing the therapy this effect can be reversed again. If, however, her menopause has already started and the ovaries no longer produce any oestrogen, the hormone continues to be formed in the fatty tissue — but even this process can be blocked with medication.

In prostate cancer the elimination of testosterone formation by the testicles is the most apparent feature. As an alternative to removal of the testicles, their deactivation by medication is therefore to be considered.

Hormone therapies attempt to eliminate the action of the sexual hormones, with corresponding side effects. In a woman the typical symptoms of menopause appear, and in a man the symptoms are similar: sleep disturbances, bouts of perspiration and headaches — but during therapy there is often great improvement. Some patients, however, suffer periodically from symptoms of depression until their body has accustomed itself to the hormone deprivation. Water retension and weight gain have also been observed.

Most of these side effects are temporary and can be handled by small adjustments in lifestyle. But if the side effects become too much of a burden, patients should talk to their doctor about taking appropriate measures.

Since the hormones introduced are not cell poisons, there are no harsh side effects as with chemotherapy, such as damage to the bone marrow and mucous membranes. However, certain anti-oestrogens used for breast cancer can, over a longer period of treatment, increase the risk for cancer in the uterus. The risk of a degenerative effect is, however, much smaller than the positive effects of the therapy and can be reduced by regular control examinations.

Curing cancer exclusively with hormone therapy is not possible as a rule. But as an additional measure, with surgery, it raises the chance of a cure, above all with breast cancer, and reduces the chance of recurrence. In the advanced state of an illness, for example with prostate cancer, hormone therapy can beneficially influence the course of the disease. Complete reversals are rare, but partial reversals or a cessation of tumour growth and metastases, can often be achieved, at least for some time. However, most tumours reach a point where they become 'hormone-deaf,' which means the tumour continues to grow despite the treatment and the continuation of the treatment no longer makes sense. In this situation, a change in hormone therapy is considered or, if all hormonal possibilities have been exhausted, chemotherapy or another measure that will mitigate the disease.

Radiation therapy (radiotherapy)

In chemotherapy the tumour cells are poisoned; in radiation therapy (US use) or radiotherapy (UK and Australian use) they are burned up. Today this combustion takes place with various rays: X-rays, gamma rays and electron beams, which all have the ability to penetrate body tissues and destroy them with heat. Unfortunately, along with this, healthy body cells are also damaged or completely incinerated. For radiologists, it is always difficult to work out a radiation plan which, while destroying the tumour, does not excessively damage healthy tissues.

As a result of radiation, besides feeling generally unwell, the patient will experience symptoms similar to sunburn: usually the skin feels irritated, becoming red and brown, and sometimes the hair falls out in the affected areas.

Stem cell therapy

The disadvantage of both chemotherapy and radiation is that healthy tissue is destroyed alongside cancerous cells, above all the blood-producing stem cells of the bone marrow, resulting in the collapse of the whole immune system. In order to be able to create fresh, healthy blood again patients need new stem cells, and for this a self-transplantation is usually undertaken. For this the patients' own stem cells are taken from their bone marrow or blood before cancer treatment, and later on, after intensive preparation, are returned in a transfusion.

It is also possible for patients to receive a stem cell transplant from a donor, preferably from their own family because then the texture characteristics will usually correspond with their own and will be better tolerated by the immune system. Recently there have also been increasingly good results with the transfer of stem cells from the blood of the umbilical cord.

Lymphoma, as well as tumours of the bone and nerve systems, are among the most common diseases in which the patient's own stem cells are transplanted.

Surgery

The surgical removal of a tumour can be done in many different ways, depending on the type and state of the tumour: from keyhole surgery all the way to
amputation. Tumours can appear anywhere in the body, in places, for example in the brain, where the surgeon has limited access or no access at all. Radiation or chemotherapy help in such cases. These two methods are also frequently used when a tumour has to be made smaller before the operation can take place. Conversely, a cancerous tumour whose complete removal is not possible can first be reduced in size surgically, in order to improve the chances of a cure with later radiation or chemotherapy.

Complementary therapies

Enzyme therapy

For some time now, researchers and physicians have found hopeful support for cancer treatment in enzyme therapies. Above all, the combination of the body's own enzymes has led to new discoveries in combating the growth of tumours. It is possible to significantly slow down the growth of cancer cells with a mix of different enzymes, and either delay or completely prevent the formation of metastases.

High dosage mixtures of enzymes are used to support other treatments during practically all phases of a tumour, above all in conjunction with radiation and chemotherapy. Clinical studies in Germany and worldwide have scientifically documented the effectiveness of enzyme therapies.

Homeopathy

Despite numerous attacks from conventional medical circles, many people have faith in homeopathy, particularly in France and Germany. Homeopathy was founded in the eighteenth century by the German physician Samuel Hahnemann. Its healing principle is based on the axiom: 'Treat like with like.' Homeopathic remedies are prescribed to strengthen the immune system and as a result to develop the self-healing powers of the patient, in this way leading to recovery. Recently, in the treatment of cancer, reports about successes achieved by homeopathic methods have been increasing.

At the beginning of every homeopathic treatment, a careful recall takes place, in which the doctor questions the patient about the history of their illness. This conversation between doctor and patient is much more intensive than one that takes place in a conventional consultation, even the descriptions of dreams, states of anxiety and moods become part of the diagnosis. The homeopath first focuses on the actual pain, then on the whole body, then finally he attempts to grasp hold of the patient's state of soul and whole personality.

Then follows the most difficult part of a homeopathic treatment: from the history of the illness and his own impressions of the patient, the physician must pinpoint the characteristic nature of the patient by means of trying to surmise his individual being — a proceeding which goes beyond the causal-analytical thinking of conventional medicine. With his intelligence and intuition an experienced homeopath discovers symptoms which he compares with the special qualities of certain remedies — plant and animal substances, minerals and metals — in order to choose the appropriate preparation.

These homeopathic medicines are taken in the form of little pellets (globuli) or drops. They are highly diluted using a process called 'potentization,' in which the original substance is shaken up, mixed and diluted ever more. This is in accordance with the homeopathic rule that the medications work more strongly the more they are diluted. The starting substance can usually no longer be detected, even in a medium potency, which brings about the criticism that homeopathy is ineffective. Most people do not take this conflict very seriously, since a lack of detection by scientific means is not the same as a lack of effectiveness.

Although there is no single method of treatment for cancer in the different schools of homeopathy, there have been some remarkable stories of cures in the last ten years. Serious homeopaths, however, always point out that the reasons for the remission of tumours are mostly unexplainable and that complete cures happen only rarely. It is also interesting that documented cures are more often ascribed to charismatic doctors than to the method as such.

Similar to traditional Chinese medicine (TCM) the homeopathic approach to cancer is based on a fundamental disturbance of the human life forces. As a rule, the younger the patient, the more localized the tumour, the slower its growth, the greater the chances are to successfully treat carcinoma by homeopathic means. But numerous cases have also been reported in which old people with metastases have reacted positively to a well-chosen homeopathic medication. On the whole, however, the successes of homeopathy for treating cancer are modest, which may also be due to the fact that the majority of patients only seek help from a homeopath when they are already in an advanced to hopeless state of illness.

Hyperthermia (heat therapy)

In recent years cancer treatments have been extended to include an increasingly important method: hyperthermia, in which cancer cells are destroyed by overheating. This approach is based on the knowledge that tumour tissue is especially sensitive to heat. In the temperature range of 40–42°C (104–107.5°F) cell membranes are damaged and the shock arising from the heat brings about changes in the cells, which enable the body's own defense system to better recognize and combat them. This effect caused by heat also makes the tumour tissue much more sensitive to the cytostatics used in chemotherapy and radiation. The effectiveness can even be doubled by the combination of both these procedures.

Healthy body cells are not damaged at these temperatures. However, the procedure is costly, involving microwaves, radio waves, infrared radiation and ultrasound.

Hyperthermia can lead to remission or to healing of a carcinoma and the metastases. Primary tumours can often be so reduced in size that surgery or other therapies are made possible. Our experience is that at least half of all cancer patients could benefit from heat therapy. In combination with other therapies the partial or even complete remission of a tumour can be achieved. Serious side effects do not occur with hyperthermia, however the increase in body temperature leads to a considerable burden on the heart and circulation. Therefore hyperthermia is often not appropriate for older or weaker patients.

Mistletoe therapy

Mistletoe therapy is the most important and most frequently used complementary treatment for cancer in Germany. It originated in anthroposophical medicine. Today in Germany it is used in two thirds of patients as a supplement to the standard 'steel, ray and chemo' methods. We have given a detailed description of this method in the main portion of this book, as well as discussing the important possibility of it providing a preventative inoculation against cancer.

Phytotherapy

The medical science of plants (phytotherapy) belongs to the very oldest medical systems. It has been practised in all the world's cultures and makes use of the whole plant or its parts, such as the stems, blossoms, leaves, fruits and roots. Plant substances have been used in many ways: as an extract, boiled down as a concentrate, as a cold water extract, as an addition to food and as a dried powder. The active plant substances also provide their healing power in the form of pills and tinctures, compresses, salves and oils, even as injections and infusions. Phytotherapy is often confused with homeopathy, with which it is related in a certain way, because plant preparations play a decisive and significant part in both forms of treatment.

When properly selected, phytotherapy can also be useful with cancer, above all to support the standard methods of 'steel, ray and chemo.' In traditional Chinese medicine (TCM), the medical science of plants plays an especially important part in curing cancer patients.

Plant medical science is very much based on experience, which is often doubted by scientists and researchers. In Christian cultural circles plant medicine was developed primarily in monasteries, always in line with the traditional folk belief that there is a plant to cure every illness. Phytotherapy has become more popular in recent years because many people mistrust highly-specialized conventional medicines and their many side effects, and are turning towards gentler means of treatment. However the medical authorities (and the pharmaceutical industry) are constantly trying to tighten the rules on the distribution of plant medications.

Plants contain many active ingredients which serve to heal illnesses. However it must not be forgotten that plants can also be extremely poisonous (e.g. foxglove, opium poppy), therefore one must be extremely careful when preparing any self-treatments!

The use of plant remedies as a supportive measure against cancer must always be discussed with an experienced doctor.

Self-regulation

Self-regulation is an extraordinarily effective method, in which cancer patients can quite consciously develop their self-healing forces in order to subdue the illness. Because cancer is more than 'just' a tumour that appears somewhere in the body; it is a condition that affects the whole person, including his soul. Of course one must aim to treat the illness with the appropriate therapies and medications, but perhaps the strongest healing factor lies within the cancer patients. If they become resigned and lose faith in themselves, then even the best doctors and medications can hardly help. Therefore it's very hard to understand why modern medicine makes little use of forces which can be called upon without financial costs.

Fortunately, ever more doctors today are remembering the traditional knowledge of the wholeness of the human being. One-sided treatment on the exclusively physical level is insufficient since it ignores the connection with soul and spirit. Holistic healing is based on the spirituality of the human being and does not separate illnesses into ailments of the body or of the soul, but always looks upon the person as a unity of body and soul. It consequently tries to perceive the cause of the illness in its totality and to pursue the process of healing on all levels.

Today no one has doubts about this close connection between body and soul, even though there is much our understanding still cannot grasp. And it is believed that the conscious development of our self-healing forces can contribute considerably towards overcoming cancer. Conversely one also knows that the constant fear of getting cancer (carcinophobia) is likely to one day lead to its outbreak.

In cancer treatment the return to one's own life forces has been given the somewhat stilted name of 'self-regulation.' What is meant by this is that patients are returning to their own life rhythm, consciously reducing daily stresses and taking responsibility for their own life, with all its joys and tears, its feelings and longings.

Dr Ronald Grossarth-Maticek investigated the significance of self-regulation for cancer patients, with groundbreaking discoveries and results. In his great study of over 10,000 cancer patients in an advanced state of the disease, he proved that the more strongly marked the self-regulation of those affected, the longer they survived the disease, regardless of the particular therapy being used. However, if at the same time there followed a treatment with mistletoe preparations, then the survival time again rose significantly — on average the patients lived two years longer than patients who weren't treated with mistletoe therapy. The study also showed that those patients who had undergone mistletoe therapy also improved their self-regulation.

Meanwhile a special training programme has been created that helps the patient to develop the ability to self-regulate in a purposeful way. This course works above all else on their basic attitude towards life, the balance between intellect and feelings, the individual's strengths and weaknesses and proper moderation in life. In order for patients to overcome step-by-step what determines their life externally and find their way back to their inner selves again, they must focus consciously on factors which can strengthen their inner forces. These include removal of stress, good diet, the transformation of destructive emotions — dealing with insults, soul injuries and grief — as well as re-establishing a balanced life rhythm.

It has been proved that cancer patients can considerably lessen their suffering with improved self-regulation. But this method helps not only in existing cases, but also as a preventative measure; it appears that the more self-determined and balanced people are, the less their danger of contracting cancer. In the end self-regulation depends on the ability to transform negative forces — dissatisfaction, rage, resignation, envy, bitterness — there are powerful energies contained in our emotions. The conscious return to a self-determined ego transforms these energies and uses them for one's own well-being. The unfettered forces that drive the unchecked growth of cancer cells can be transformed: self-regulation of the human being shows the way to do so.

This is wonderful news for the cancer patient. Although the deep connections between self-regulation and active mistletoe substances have not yet been entirely established, the investigation proved that the conscious structuring of one's own life, self-confidence, positivity, happiness and looking after oneself all help to prolong the life of the cancer patient. Of course, it is down to the patient to make this effort, but it is also sensible to seek the help of a doctor or on experienced therapist.

Shamanism

Self-regulation is not only in accord with the healing principles of anthroposophical medicine but surprisingly enough with those of the oldest healing method we know about: shamanism.

In all the early cultures of the world a treasury of experience was amassed in which knowledge of human spirituality, along with a recognition of the healing powers of nature — the elements of earth, water, fire and air, as well as those of the plants, animals and stones — was contained. In this all-embracing worldview, one proceeds from the assumption that everything is alive and an illness appears whenever a person's relationship to other creatures, to nature or to the cosmic order has fallen out of balance.

Shamans have the ability to connect the spirit of a human being with the spiritual forces in nature and thereby effect the healing of an illness. Shamans also work with herbs, with tried medical traditions, with ritual treatments such as drums, songs and the laying on of hands, but in a deeper sense they are spiritual healers, who aim to bring sick people into harmony with themselves and with creation once again. The shamanistic healing concept is the transformation of the negative energies which have caused an illness into new, positive energies. Patients recover because, with the help of the shaman, they strengthen their own self-healing forces.

Such methods may make some people smile, but the healing successes of shamans are incontestable. At some German university clinics various shamanistic methods are currently being scientifically followed and investigated. And since 1980 the World Health Organization (WHO) has recognized shamanism to be just as significant as conventional medical therapies for treating psychosomatic illnesses.

We do not want to raise any false hopes with this description of shamanistic treatment, but solely to point out the similarities to the proven success of self-regulation. Taking a holistic view of cancer and developing self-healing forces appears to give a good chance of recovery. However it would be short-sighted for anyone suffering from cancer to detour conventional medicine and seek help exclusively from a shaman who will not tolerate any additional treatment, and whose expensive promises of a cure may unfortunately burst like soap bubbles.

Traditional Chinese medicine (TCM)

According to TCM doctrine there are three factors which promote the formation of cancer:

Food assimilation problems — caused by bad diet, remains of
     medication in the body, environmental poisons.
Stressed mucous membranes — caused by chronic inflammations,
     psychological trauma, menstrual cycle disturbances.
Qi (energy flow) stagnation — blockages due to immune
     problems, conflicts, accidents, psychological problems.

In traditional Chinese medicine cancer is interpreted as stagnation
of the blood and of *qi*. The cancer cells themselves are considered
to be weak and to abhor three things: warmth, hunger and oxygen.
The cancer therapy of TCM is always concerned with providing
the patient with sufficient warmth as well as taming malignant
cells by giving patients appropriate nourishment and an intensive
supply of oxygen.

Along with this, *qigong*, a special form of movement and
breathing practice which originated in China, has proved helpful
as a supplement to the necessary medical treatments. *Qigong* is
the combination of three elements: conscious breathing, slow and
calm movements and the concentration on both of these and/or
on particular areas of the body. Besides a salutary relaxation and
psychological stabilization, these techniques improve circulation
and oxygen supply to the body.

In particular, a special form of *qigong*, *Fan Teng Gong*, brings
about a strong activation of the energy centre in the human being.
After a relatively short time, patients feel a strong inner upwelling
of heat: in this way cancer cells are directly attacked and at the
same time the body develops the capacity to heal itself.

In TCM bodily perception is an important learning process
that sensitizes people to negative developments in the body,
because according to Chinese understanding, cancer arises due
to insufficient control over cell growth. Through inner calm,
regular breathing and a harmonious inner balance, cell rhythm
can be stabilized: in this the Chinese see an effective measure
of prevention. *Qigong* calms the human being, regulates the
breathing and thereby strengthens the *yin*, the inner structure of
order.

In China diet also plays an important role in the treatment of cancer. Food substances from the sea that contain iodine, such as seaweed and algae, are supposed to be very effective, above all for treating lymphoma. The tree mushroom is said to have a positive effect on the lungs, and a soup can be made from licorice and mung beans which is supposed to mitigate the side effects of chemotherapy and radiation.

On the whole, diet recommendations vary according to the individual's particular digestive situation, but the following is generally true:

1. Eat as many fresh vegetables as possible, not overcooked, only steamed.
2. Eat few eggs (albumin) and no dairy products.
3. Avoid processed foods because of additives in meats, preservatives and artificial colouring.
4. Drink warm tea regularly.

Traditional Chinese medicine has great faith in phytotherapy; it recognises 3000 different plants and connects a third of them directly or indirectly with tumour treatments. While the plants have no direct effect on a tumour, they strengthen the resistance of the organism against the degenerate cells. The plants recommended by the TCM are first boiled down, then the decoction is taken in little sips, spreading the healing impulses regularly over the whole day. TCM doctors warn that their healing herbs are not suitable for self-medication since they are not freely sold, and it isn't possible to create effective remedies without having professional knowledge.

Acupuncture also plays a certain part in TCM cancer therapy, and for that an experienced professional is certainly needed. It is about ten times more expensive than phytotherapy. Besides which, an acupuncture treatment has a lesser long-term effect than a daily dosage of herbal treatments.

The feeling of nausea following chemotherapy can be greatly reduced by acupuncture treatment just before the chemotherapy.

It is even better to leave the acupuncture needles in for some time during the chemo treatment. However the significance of acupuncture in the treatment of tumours is much less than TCM therapy based on plants.

According to TCM there are currents of energy in every human being. In 'acupuncture massage' (without needles) the course of these currents (meridians) is followed and stimulated with a little rod. This procedure has very much proven itself in the treatment of painful scar tissue and for the healing of deep-seated wounds. According to the teaching of TCM a scar creates a *qi* blockage which, if not treated, can lead to a long-lasting interruption of the energy flow.

TCM knows of no procedure in which tumour cells are directly destroyed or in which growth is checked. The aim is rather to strengthen the organism in its defense against cancer cells. In that way TCM can supplement conventional medicine, above all in the areas of aftercare, dealing with the illness and secondary prevention (avoiding recurrences).

Therefore in cancer therapy conventional medicine such as chemotherapy and TCM can go hand in hand. TCM does not regard itself as an alternative to the methods of modern medicine, but as a supplement to it. In China, western therapies are also used in the fight against cancer tumours.

Contact Addresses

Anthroposophic clinics and practitioners' associations

Great Britain

Park Attwood Clinic
Trimpley, Bewdley,
Worcestershire DY12 1RE
Tel: +44 (0)1299 861 444
Web: www.parkattwood.org
Email: info@parkattwood.org

General practitioners:
A current list can be found on the Anthroposophic Health and
Social Care website: http://ahasc.org.uk/directory/

United States

Physicians' Association for Anthroposophic Medicine (PAAM)
123 Geddes Avenue
Ann Arbor, MI 48104
Tel: +1 734 930 9462
Web: www.paam.net
Email: paam@anthroposophy.org

Canada

Canadian Anthroposophical Medicine Association
7-9100 Bathurst Street, Suite 2
Hesperus Community, Thornhill
Ontario L4J 8C7
Tel: +1 905 882 4949

Australia

Australian Anthroposophic Medicine Association
Web: http://www.aamaanthro.com
Email: info@AAMAanthro.com.au

New Zealand

Anthroposophical Society in New Zealand
Sue Simpson, General Secretary
PO Box 8279, Havelock
Tel: +64 (0)6 8776656
Web: www.anthroposophy.org.nz

South Africa

Syringa Holistic Health Centre
Wembley Road 4
Plumstead 7800, Cape Town
Tel: + 27 (0)21 762 2364
          + 27 (0)21 762 0862
Web: www.syringahealth.co.za
Email: syringacentre@netpoint.co.za

Index

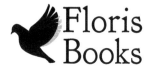**Floris Books**

For news on all our **latest books,**
and to receive **exclusive discounts,**
join our mailing list at:

florisbooks.co.uk

Plus subscribers get a **FREE** book
with every online order!

Lightning Source UK Ltd.
Milton Keynes UK
UKHW020854150322
400051UK00005B/70